CHANGE YOURSELF, CHANGE THE WORLD

HARNESS YOUR SEXUAL ENERGY FOR ACTIVATION

FLOYD J SANDERS

Disclaimer:

The content presented in "Change Yourself, Change the World: Harness Your Sexual Energy for Activation" is intended for informational and educational purposes only. The views, opinions, and recommendations expressed in this book are those of the author and do not necessarily reflect the views of the publisher.

Readers are advised to use their discretion and judgment when considering the information provided in this book. The author is not a licensed medical professional, and the book does not constitute professional advice in the fields of medicine, psychology, or any other related disciplines. It is crucial for individuals to consult with qualified professionals for personalized advice tailored to their specific circumstances.

The book explores topics related to celibacy, abstinence, and the potential impact of sexual energy on various aspects of life. While the author has made efforts to present well-researched and evidence-based information, readers are encouraged to conduct their own research and seek guidance from qualified experts to make informed decisions.

The author and the publisher are not responsible for any actions taken by individuals based on the information presented in this book. Readers are solely responsible for the consequences of their choices and actions.

By reading this book, readers acknowledge and accept that the content is not a substitute for professional advice, and they should consult with appropriate professionals for guidance on matters related to their health, well-being, and personal development.

The publisher disclaims any liability or responsibility for errors, omissions, or inaccuracies in the content and for any consequences arising from the use or interpretation of the information provided in this book.

Contents

Introduction

Throughout history, celibacy and abstinence have held significant roles in various cultures and religions. These practices have been linked to spiritual, philosophical, and moral beliefs, often viewed as pathways to higher levels of consciousness or acts of self-discipline and restraint.

In ancient Greece, celibacy was promoted by certain philosophical schools like the Pythagoreans and Stoics, who believed in restraining desires for intellectual and moral advancement. The Essenes, a Jewish sect during Jesus' time, practiced celibacy and communal living as part of their spiritual pursuits. Hinduism has a longstanding tradition of asceticism and renunciation, valuing celibacy for those seeking spiritual enlightenment, as seen in the practice of Brahmacharya. Buddhism emphasizes celibacy as one of the monastic precepts, aiming to eliminate worldly distractions and attachments. In Christianity, celibacy has been upheld by specific religious orders and clergy as a means of dedicating oneself entirely to God and spiritual service. Within Islam, certain Sufi orders promote celibacy or abstaining from worldly desires to achieve closeness to God.

During the Enlightenment period, philosophers such as Immanuel Kant and Arthur Schopenhauer discussed celibacy and abstinence as moral choices and methods to attain higher ethical ideals.

Immanuel Kant, a German philosopher renowned for his emphasis on reason and moral duty, viewed celibacy and abstinence as displays of self-discipline and moral fortitude. He argued that by restraining desires and prioritizing moral principles, individuals could align their actions with universal ethical laws.

Arthur Schopenhauer, another influential

philosopher of the time, saw celibacy and abstinence as ways to transcend desires and find inner peace and fulfillment. He believed that renouncing sensual pleasures and worldly attachments could lead to a deeper understanding of oneself and the nature of reality.

Henry David Thoreau, an American transcendentalist philosopher, expressed his support for celibacy and abstinence in his famous work "Walden." Thoreau's book recounts his experience of living a simple, self-sufficient life in a cabin near Walden Pond. For Thoreau, celibacy was a means to eliminate distractions and concentrate on individual reflection, spiritual growth, and a deeper connection with nature.

These philosophical perspectives during the Enlightenment period sparked intellectual discourse on the merits of celibacy and abstinence. They reflected a broader questioning of societal norms and explored alternative ways of living that prioritized personal introspection, moral integrity, and the pursuit of higher truths.

The sexual revolution of the 20th century brought about a significant change in societal attitudes towards celibacy and abstinence, breaking away from the traditional associations of these practices with moral obligations or religious mandates.

During this era, the dominant cultural narrative prioritized exploring one's sexuality, liberating oneself from sexual repression, and embracing individual desires. Celibacy and abstinence were often regarded as outdated or restrictive ideas that hindered personal fulfillment and sexual liberation. However, in recent times, there has been a noticeable resurgence of interest in celibacy and abstinence as lifestyle choices. People are increasingly exploring these practices influenced by various factors, including concerns about health, personal growth, and the environment.

Celibacy and abstinence are viewed by some as ways to maintain both physical and emotional well-being. By refraining from sexual activities, individuals prioritize their mental and physical health, avoiding the potential risks associated with casual encounters or sexually transmitted infections. Additionally, abstaining from sexual relationships allows us to focus on personal growth, self-discovery, and pursuing other aspects of their lives without distractions. The consideration of environmental concerns has also led to a reevaluation of celibacy and abstinence. By reducing sexual partners or practicing celibacy, we can minimize their carbon footprint and contribute to a more sustainable lifestyle by avoiding the potential negative impacts of multiple sexual relationships on the environment.

This renewed interest in celibacy and abstinence highlights the various motivations and factors behind these choices. It signifies a shift towards embracing individual agency and recognizing that celibacy and abstinence can be conscious lifestyle decisions aligned with personal values, well-being, and the pursuit of a fulfilling life beyond societal norms.

Throughout history, many thought leaders have made similar points, emphasizing the pursuit of higher spiritual or moral ideals through renouncing worldly desires, the belief that celibacy and abstinence can lead to increased self-discipline, focus, and personal growth, and the view of celibacy and abstinence as acts of devotion or enlightenment. They also stressed the importance of community support and guidance in navigating these practices. Exploring specific thought leaders and their teachings can offer a deeper understanding of the diverse perspectives throughout history.

If every man and woman committed to practicing intermittent celibacy and abstinence, it could potentially have significant impacts on various aspects of society, including reducing crime, STD transmission, population growth, and individual personal-spiritual development. This exploration delves into the potential social, economic, and global effects.

Chapter 1:
Decreasing Crime

Reducing sexual activity through celibacy and abstinence can potentially contribute to lowering the number of unplanned pregnancies. As our generation has experienced, unplanned pregnancies, especially when we are not emotionally or financially prepared, lead to unstable family situations.

Thousands of studies have demonstrated that unstable family environments, characterized by high levels of stress, financial difficulties, and limited parental support, can increase the risk of criminal behavior in children. Our parents and we, fully possessed by the free love movement as well as the free use of drugs, alcohol, and other substances, lived very indulgent lives, and our generations have paid the price. Our generations are a living testament to this.

Now, it's not too late for us to learn from our past, turn pain into wisdom, and chart out a new future for our children and grandchildren by tearing down the old system of overindulgence. We can yet choose celibacy and abstinence. We can consciously decide to avoid engaging in sexual activities that may result in unplanned pregnancies and stress this to our children and grandchildren. This can promote more intentional family planning, allowing children and children's children to establish stable family structures when they feel ready and capable of providing a nurturing environment for their children. Stable family environments, in turn, can have a positive impact on child development, reducing the likelihood of delinquency or criminal behavior in the future. We yet have it within our power to pave a brighter future for children.

It is crucial to acknowledge that the correlation between unstable family structures and crime rates is complex and affected by different social and economic factors. Although reducing unplanned pregnancies through celibacy and abstinence might indirectly contribute to lowering crime rates, it is merely one component of a comprehensive strategy to tackle crime and foster societal welfare. Other elements like educational access, socioeconomic opportunities, community support, and effective social policies also play vital roles in preventing crime.

Engaging in celibacy and abstinence can offer us the chance to prioritize personal development, education, and career aspirations. These factors have been linked to a decreased likelihood of participating in criminal activities. Let's explore how celibacy and abstinence can play a role in preventing crime through personal growth.

Sexual Abstinence and Celibacy and Personal Growth

By refraining from sexual activities for periods of time, we can devote our time, energy, and focus to personal advancement. This may involve pursuing spiritual development, education, acquiring new skills, enjoying hobbies, and cultivating a strong sense of self.

Personal growth nurtures self-confidence, a positive self-image, and a sense of purpose, diminishing the inclination to partake in criminal behavior. Our generation can prioritize our education and seize opportunities for learning and skill-building. Education provides us with knowledge, critical thinking abilities, and improved job prospects, which can contribute to economic stability and discourage involvement in criminal activities driven by desperation or limited opportunities.

Choosing celibacy and abstinence allows us to dedicate more time and mental energy towards our career goals. By focusing on professional growth, we can improve our skills, advance in our careers, and achieve financial stability. Having stable employment and economic well-being also serves as protective factors against involvement in criminal activities.

Emotional stability serves as a solid foundation for decision-making, as it enables individuals to approach choices with clarity and rationality. When emotions are in check, people can carefully weigh the pros and cons of different options and make decisions that align with their long-term goals and values. This ability to make well-informed choices reduces the likelihood of succumbing to impulsive behaviors driven by momentary desires or temporary satisfaction.

Moreover, celibacy and abstinence contribute to improved self-control. Engaging in sexual relationships can sometimes lead to impulsive actions driven by desire, passion, or societal pressure. However, by practicing celibacy or abstinence, we develop the ability to manage our impulses and resist immediate gratification. This heightened self-control allows us to exercise discipline and restraint in various aspects of life, ultimately leading to more balanced and thoughtful decision-making overall.

Additionally, emotional stability gained through celibacy and abstinence plays a crucial role in resolving conflicts. Relationships, especially intimate ones, can often result in disagreements and conflicts. Yet, when we are emotionally stable, we can approach these conflicts with a calm and rational mindset, seeking understanding and resolution instead of resorting to aggressive or confrontational behavior. Emotional well-being provides the necessary foundation to peacefully navigate conflicts and find mutually satisfying resolutions, which in turn fosters healthier relationships and stronger interpersonal connections.

Celibacy and abstinence can positively impact emotional well-being by avoiding the potential negative consequences of casual or unhealthy sexual relationships. By promoting emotional stability, these practices enable us to make better decisions, exercise self-control, and resolve conflicts more effectively. The resulting emotional well-being provides a solid basis for a healthier and more fulfilling life, ultimately enhancing overall happiness and satisfaction.

Additionally, choosing to occasionally abstaining from sexual relationships can lead us to prioritize building healthy and meaningful connections with others, creating a supportive network that discourages criminal involvement and fosters positive social interactions.

Another significant advantage of occasionally from sexual relationships is the opportunity to foster connections that go beyond physical attraction or sexual desire. These relationships are built on a strong foundation of mutual respect, emotional intimacy, and shared interests. By prioritizing these qualities, we can form lasting bonds that promote personal growth, emotional well-being, and overall life satisfaction.

Furthermore, by prioritizing the establishment of healthy connections, we can create a supportive network that discourages engagement in criminal activities. Strong relationships founded on trust and respect provide us with a sense of belonging and social support, reducing feelings of isolation and vulnerability. This support system acts as a protective factor, offering guidance, encouragement, and accountability, which can effectively deter us from participating in criminal behaviors.

In addition, choosing to abstain from sexual relationships allows us to prioritize their personal values and moral principles when interacting with others. This intentional decision enables them to align our actions with our beliefs and promotes ethical behavior within our relationships. Surrounding ourselves with like-minded others who share similar values helps us create a positive social environment that encourages integrity, honesty, and compassion.

Moreover, focusing on building healthy and meaningful connections can have a positive impact on social interactions and community engagement. By investing time and energy into nurturing relationships, we can actively participate in community activities, volunteer work, and support networks. This involvement fosters a sense of social responsibility, promotes positive change, and contributes to a more cohesive and supportive community.

While celibacy and abstinence can contribute to personal development and factors known to reduce criminal activities, it is important to recognize that crime is influenced by various complex social, economic, and individual factors. Comprehensive crime prevention efforts should involve a combination of strategies, including community support, education, access to resources, and addressing the root causes of criminal behavior. Fewer sexual encounters, which can result from practicing celibacy and abstinence, can potentially contribute to a decrease in instances of sexual assault and harassment.

Here's how celibacy and abstinence may play a role in reducing these forms of misconduct. By practicing celibacy or abstinence at the beginning of a relationship, we can consciously avoid engaging in sexual behaviors that might end result in emotional trauma. This emphasizes the importance of clear and explicit consent in any sexual encounter. Consent is crucial to ensuring that all parties involved are fully willing and actively participating in any sexual activity. Understanding and respecting boundaries are essential aspects of fostering a culture of consent and preventing sexual assault.

Celibacy and abstinence encourage us to establish and assert our personal boundaries regarding sexual activities. This promotes the idea that everyone has the right to determine their comfort levels and what they are willing to engage in. By practicing celibacy and abstinence, we can develop a strong sense of personal agency and boundary-setting, which contributes to a healthier and more respectful approach to intimate relationships.

Occasionally, opting out of sexual encounters entirely reduces the chances of finding oneself in potentially risky or dangerous situations. Engaging in consensual sexual activity necessitates trust, communication, and mutual understanding. However, in certain cases where consent is ignored or violated, sexual assault and harassment can occur. By refraining from sexual encounters, people can minimize their exposure to these risks. Celibacy and abstinence can also contribute to challenging and dismantling rape culture.

By actively choosing not to partake in sexual activities for periods of time, we can help change societal attitudes that may perpetuate or normalize harmful behaviors. Promoting respect, consent, and healthy relationships through personal choices can contribute to a wider cultural shift in preventing sexual assault and harassment. While celibacy and abstinence can aid in reducing instances of sexual assault and harassment, it is important to acknowledge that addressing these issues requires comprehensive approaches involving education, consent culture, and supportive systems to create safer environments for everyone.

Chapter 2: Preventing the Transmission of STDs

Celibacy and abstinence offer us a complete solution to eliminating the risk of transmitting and/or contracting sexually transmitted diseases (STDs), resulting in a significant reduction in their spread in our population. How do celibacy and abstinence contribute to preventing the transmission of STDs?

By refraining from sexual activities for periods of time, we can completely eliminate the possibility of direct STD transmission through sexual contact during those periods of time. Since most STDs are primarily transmitted through sexual intercourse or intimate activities, celibacy and abstinence provide a reliable method of preventing such infections and improving our sexual health. We have to severe our ties with the free love culture over indulgence culture if we are to survive.

With our generation acting as a barrier against infection by practicing celibacy and abstinence, we act as a shield against exposure to STDs and transmission. By reducing our sexual encounters and refraining from intimate activities for periods, during these times, we can prevent the exchange of bodily fluids that can carry STDs, like semen, vaginal fluids, and blood. This effectively eliminates the primary mode of transmission for many sexually transmitted infections.

It is important to note that many STDs can be transmitted even when individuals show no symptoms. By practicing celibacy and abstinence, our generation can ensure that we improve and preserve our sexual health and do not unknowingly transmit STDs or contract them from asymptomatic carriers. While condoms are an effective method of reducing the risk of STD transmission, they are not completely fool-proof. By practicing celibacy and abstinence, we eliminate the need to rely solely on the correct and consistent use of condoms, further minimizing the risk of STD transmission. We have paid a high price for free love and over indulgence, thereby coming to the great understanding: There is NO such thing as free love.

Beyond the prevention of STDs, celibacy and abstinence contribute to overall sexual health and well-being. By avoiding multiple sexual partners, we reduce their exposure to potential infections and complications associated with certain STDs, such as infertility, cervical cancer (linked to Human Papillomavirus, HPV), or long-term consequences of untreated infections. However, it is important to emphasize that even though we may practice celibacy and abstinence, we should continue to engage in regular health screenings and consult healthcare professionals about the impact of previous sexual activity and how those past choices may be impacting us today to catch potential health risks before they become life-threatening. Open communication and education about sexual health remain crucial for maintaining well-being.

How Promoting Responsible Sexual Behavior Can Prevent the Transmission of STDs

Promoting responsible sexual behavior, including the choice to abstain from sexual activity, plays a vital role in curbing the spread of sexually transmitted diseases (STDs) and protecting us. Here's how the promotion of responsible sexual behavior can help prevent the transmission of STDs.

Encouraging abstinence as a primary prevention strategy is highly effective against STDs. By promoting abstaining from sexual activity, especially if not in a mutually monogamous and committed relationship, the risk of exposure to STDs is significantly reduced. Educating us on risk reduction through promoting responsible sexual behavior involves comprehensive sexual education that includes information about STDs, their modes of transmission, and prevention methods. By raising awareness about the risks associated with unprotected sexual activity and the importance of not putting complete trust in using barrier methods like condoms, we can make informed decisions to protect themselves and others.

Encouraging responsible sexual behavior is crucial in promoting the our well-being. Regular testing for STDs is especially important for sexually active individuals as it helps in the early identification and treatment of STDs, ultimately preventing their further transmission. Additionally, practicing abstinence during the waiting period for test results can further reduce the risk of potential transmission. By promoting healthy relationships through open communication, mutual consensual abstinence or celibacy, and the use of alternative non-penetrative, non-body fluid exchanging sex methods like some forms of tantric sex, we can minimize the likelihood of engaging in high-risk behaviors that can lead to transmission of STDs.

Creating an environment where we feel comfortable discussing sexual health and seeking help when needed is also a part of promoting responsible sexual behavior. By reducing the stigma and shame associated with STDs, we can encourage people to seek timely testing, treatment, and support, thereby preventing the further spread of infections.

Comprehensive Sexual Education

Advocating responsible sexual behavior, including abstinence as a valid choice, empowers us to make informed decisions about their sexual health. This empowerment plays a significant role in reducing the transmission of STDs, protecting our well-being, and safeguarding public health. By providing comprehensive education and support, we can understand the potential risks and consequences associated with sexual activity, as well as the various preventive measures available to protect themselves and others.

Comprehensive sexual education programs, including alternatives to penetrative or oral sex, are essential in empowering us to make informed decisions about their sexual health. These programs go beyond solely focusing on abstinence and instead prioritize the dissemination of accurate and evidence-based information. By covering topics like safe sex practices, contraception, regular testing, and communication skills, comprehensive sexual education equips us with the knowledge and tools to navigate their sexual lives responsibly.

Accurate information about the risks of STDs and prevention methods is particularly crucial in sexual education. Such education helps us understand the potential consequences of our actions and empowers us to take proactive steps to protect our own well-being and that of our partners. By providing comprehensive information about STDs, we are better equipped to assess the risks associated with various sexual activities and make informed choices about their sexual behavior.

Furthermore, comprehensive sexual education programs promote a holistic understanding of sexual health by addressing a wide range of topics. By covering safe sex practices and esoteric sex practices, we can learn about the effective use of touch and contraceptives, the importance of regular testing for STDs, and the significance of open and honest communication with our partners to expand intimacy beyond physical sexual contact. These skills and knowledge not only contribute to the prevention of STDs but also foster healthier relationships, promote consent, and improve overall sexual well-being.

By moving beyond a narrow focus on abstinence-only education, comprehensive sexual education recognizes the diverse needs, beliefs, options, and circumstances available to us to enhance the sexual experience beyond physical contact. It acknowledges that abstinence is one choice among many and provides us with a broader understanding of our options. This inclusive approach allows us to make decisions that align with our personal values and circumstances while still being well-informed about the potential risks and consequences associated with sexual activity.

It is important to acknowledge and promote abstinence as a valid choice within comprehensive sexual education. By presenting abstinence as one option among many, we can make decisions that align with our personal values, beliefs, and circumstances. Highlighting the potential benefits of abstinence, such as avoiding unintended pregnancies, reducing the risk of STDs, and maintaining emotional well-being, encourages us to consider this option as part of our sexual decision-making.

When abstinence is presented as a valid choice, we can consider the potential benefits it offers. Abstinence provides a reliable method for avoiding unintended pregnancies, as it eliminates the risk of conception altogether. Additionally, choosing abstinence significantly reduces the risk of contracting sexually transmitted diseases (STDs), as sexual activity is the primary mode of transmission for many infections.

By highlighting these benefits, we are encouraged to carefully consider abstinence as part of our sexual decision-making process.

Furthermore, promoting abstinence recognizes the importance of emotional well-being alongside physical health. Engaging in sexual activity is an intimate experience that can have profound emotional consequences. Abstinence allows us to prioritize our emotional well-being by avoiding potential complexities and complications that can arise from sexual relationships. It offers the opportunity to develop a strong sense of self, establish personal boundaries, and focus on personal growth without the added complexities that sexual activity may bring.

Open Communication as a Means to Promote Responsible Sexual Behavior

To promote responsible sexual behavior, it is vital to establish a transparent and accepting conversation about sexuality, relationships, and sexual well-being. This creates a secure and supportive environment where we can seek information, ask questions, and address concerns without facing stigma or shame. By fostering an open dialogue, we are encouraged to explore and understand our own sexuality in a safe and non-judgmental space. This empowers us to acquire accurate and evidence-based knowledge about a persons sexual health, prior contraceptive use, consent practices, and other crucial aspects of responsible sexual behavior. Offering comprehensive sexual education enables us to make informed decisions, understand our rights and boundaries, and engage in healthy sexual practices.

Furthermore, initiating open discussions about sexuality and relationships facilitates healthier and more respectful connections. By emphasizing consent, communication, and boundaries, we can develop a deeper comprehension of the significance of mutual respect, trust, and effective communication within sexual relationships. This enables partners to navigate our desires and preferences in a consensual and mutually satisfying manner, contributing to healthier and more fulfilling connections.

Moreover, an open conversation about sexual health and relationships helps dismantle the barriers of stigma and shame often attached to these topics. By creating a secure space to express concerns, seek support, and share experiences, the culture of shame and judgment can be eradicated. This empowers us to approach our sexual health confidently, seek medical assistance when needed, and address any issues or challenges without fear of discrimination or prejudice.

In addition, open communication promotes inclusivity and the recognition of various sexual orientations, identities, and experiences. By acknowledging and respecting the diverse spectrum of sexual orientations and gender identities, we can create an environment that is all-encompassing and affirming. This fosters a sense of acceptance and value for us, regardless of our sexual orientation or gender identity, and promotes a feeling of belonging and self-acceptance.

Access to Resources and Healthcare

Access to resources and healthcare plays a critical role in empowering our generation to make responsible choices regarding our sexual health. It ensures that they have the necessary tools, information, and support to protect their well-being. Affordable and convenient access to contraceptives and condoms is of utmost importance in promoting responsible sexual behavior; however, broader than this, setting abstinence or celibacy boundaries for a period at the start of any relationship is far more crucial. The era of one-night stands must come to an end as we realize our sexual organs are far more precious than this and the cost of abusing or misusing them. A one-night stand can turn into a lifetime responsibility and mental, physical, or emotional challenges. One-night stands are very risky. By making these resources easily available, we are more than just our sex organs and are empowered to take control of our reproductive health and prevent unintended pregnancies. Affordable contraception options enable us to choose the method that aligns with their preferences and needs, promoting a sense of autonomy and informed decision-making. While I am an advocate for sex within the boundaries of marriage, monogamy, or celibacy, and abstinence in between as a means reduce or prevent transmission, I recognize that not everyone is at a level of self-control to refrain; however, while we may trust that the availability of high-quality contraception allows that allows us to engage in safer sexual practices, we must acknowledge that in the heat of the moment, bodily fluid exchanges can and do happen. Reducing the risk of sexually transmitted infections and promoting overall sexual health must be our focus rather than a fun romp.

Regular testing for sexually transmitted diseases (STDs) is a crucial aspect of responsible sexual behavior. Access to affordable and accessible testing facilities plays a vital role in early detection, treatment, and prevention of the spread of STDs. Regular testing empowers us to be aware of our own health status and that of any potential partner and to take appropriate measures to protect themselves and our partners. By ensuring that testing services are readily accessible, convenient, and affordable, we are more likely to seek timely and regular testing, contributing to overall public health by reducing the transmission of STDs.

Furthermore, providing information about local clinics, healthcare providers, and support services is essential for us to effectively address their sexual health needs and concerns. Accessible information enables us to navigate the healthcare system and identify resources that can provide the necessary care and support. By connecting with knowledgeable healthcare professionals, we can receive accurate information, guidance, and counseling tailored to their specific needs. Additionally, awareness of local clinics and support services encourages us to seek assistance in a timely manner, fostering a proactive approach to sexual health. Moreover, the adult industry must also join in by creating content that does not depict or display sexual conduct that is of a rape nature or nonconsensual sexual acts or scenes. Consent must be conveyed in the scene so as not to glamorize violent, unsafe sexual practices. Given that children now access online porn with a click of a button, just clicking a button that asks you if you are 18 is not enough. It's time for the adult film industry to catch up and become advocates.

Chapter 3:
Population Reduction

Indeed, choosing to remain celibate or abstain from sexual activity can have a positive impact on reducing unplanned pregnancies, which in turn can contribute to lower population growth rates. By abstaining from sex for periods of time, we eliminate the risk of unintended pregnancies that can occur due to contraceptive failures or inconsistent use.

Unplanned pregnancies, especially when people are not prepared or ready to become parents, can contribute to population growth. Opting for celibacy and abstinence allows us to prioritize our personal goals, education, and career aspirations, enabling us to make informed decisions about family planning. By consciously deciding when and under what circumstances to start a family, we can better manage our reproductive choices and contribute to controlling population growth.

With fewer unplanned pregnancies, we can allocate our resources, including time, finances, and emotional support, more effectively to existing children or personal endeavors. This can lead to improved access to healthcare, education, and opportunities for economic advancement, ultimately fostering a higher quality of life for us and our families. Achieving a lower population growth rate through reduced unplanned pregnancies can also contribute to environmental sustainability. As the global population continues to rise, there is increased strain on resources, heightened carbon emissions, and ecological challenges. By curbing population growth, celibacy and abstinence can help alleviate these environmental issues, promoting a more sustainable balance between human needs and the planet's resources. Abstinence and the prevention of unplanned pregnancies can indeed support planned pregnancies, as they provide us with the opportunity to make intentional decisions about starting a family and better prepare for the responsibilities that come with parenthood.

By choosing celibacy to focus on self-improvement or spiritual growth or practicing abstinence effectively, we have greater control over our reproductive choices and can actively devote more time to their existing personal endeavors. Abstinence, in particular, allows us to delay starting a family until they feel emotionally, financially, and logistically ready. It provides us with the time and space to prioritize our own personal goals, educational pursuits, career advancement, or relationship stability before embarking on the journey of parenthood. By intentionally avoiding unplanned pregnancies, can take the necessary steps to create a stable and supportive environment for their future children.

The prevention of unplanned pregnancies through abstinence allows us to plan for our pregnancies in terms of our own health and well-being. By avoiding unintended pregnancies, we can focus on optimizing our physical health, such as maintaining a balanced diet, engaging in regular exercise, and avoiding harmful substances. They can also address any underlying mental or health conditions or seek necessary therapeutic or medical interventions, ensuring that we are in the best possible condition to conceive and carry a pregnancy to term. Taking the time to prioritize our own health can contribute to healthier pregnancies and better outcomes for both the parent and the child.

By avoiding unplanned pregnancies, we have the opportunity to establish stable and supportive relationships before starting a family. They can dedicate time to building a strong foundation of trust, emotional connection, and effective communication with their partners. This ensures that we enter parenthood with a solid partnership, increasing the likelihood of successful co-parenting and a supportive environment for the child. Planning for a pregnancy allows us to create a nurturing and loving environment where we can provide the emotional, financial, and practical support needed for our children's well-being.

However, it is important to acknowledge that population growth is a multifaceted issue influenced by various factors, such as fertility rates, cultural norms, and socioeconomic conditions. While celibacy and abstinence can contribute to population reduction by decreasing unplanned pregnancies, comprehensive approaches to population control and sustainable development should also encompass access to spiritual, religious, or martial arts training for self-development and discipline, impulse and self-control training, educational opportunities, vocational training, and addressing social and economic inequalities that may contribute to risk-taking behaviors and unplanned pregnancies. Voluntary controlled population growth through celibacy and abstinence can bring several potential benefits.

Impact of Reduced Population on Resource Distribution

A reduced rate of population growth facilitates the more efficient allocation of resources, including food, water, housing, and energy. This relieves the pressure on finite resources and fosters fair access to fundamental necessities. Here's how managing population growth can positively impact resource distribution:

Decreased population growth facilitates improved allocation and distribution of food resources, relieving strain on agricultural systems and promoting sustainable and efficient production and distribution of food. This effectively tackles food scarcity, minimizes competition for limited resources, and enhances food security for our communities.

By maintaining a voluntary controlled population growth rate, we can enhance our ability to manage our water resources effectively. This enables us to implement improved practices such as sustainable usage, conservation, and fair distribution of water. Instead of concentrating populations in cities, we spread out creating smaller population concentrations, there will be less competition for water resources, guaranteeing that everyone has access to clean and an ample supply of water to meet their needs.

With a decrease in population growth and concentrations, the burden on housing and infrastructure is alleviated. This paves the way for more effective planning and implementation of housing initiatives, guaranteeing everyone can avail of secure and reasonably priced housing. Moreover, it facilitates the adequate construction and upkeep of infrastructure, encompassing transportation, sanitation, and utilities, thereby enhancing the overall living standards for everyone.

Managing voluntary participation in population growth and concentration reduction programs can play a role in promoting sustainable energy consumption. A smaller population means less need for energy resources, easing the burden on energy production and the environment. This paves the way for the advancement and acceptance of renewable energy sources, ultimately leading to a more sustainable and eco-friendly energy system.

Promoting fairness in resource access through slower population growth and by spreading population is crucial. Decreasing competition for limited resources guarantees fair and equal access to essential needs, particularly for vulnerable or marginalized communities. Ultimately, this aids in reducing socioeconomic disparities and fostering overall social well-being.

Impact of Voluntary Controlled Population Growth on Resource Management

It is crucial to acknowledge that achieving sustainable resource distribution goes beyond just controlling population growth and reducing the concentration of population. It requires comprehensive approaches that encompass sustainable resource management, technological advancements, conservation practices, and addressing socioeconomic disparities to ensure a fair and sustainable future for everyone.

Voluntary controlled population growth programs play a vital role in facilitating more manageable infrastructure development, leading to an enhanced quality of life and well-functioning urban environments.

By practicing celibacy or abstinence, we can have an impact on our transportation systems. How? Slower population growth allows for more effective planning and development of transportation systems. This enables the construction of transportation infrastructure that adequately caters to the population's needs, such as roads, public transportation networks, and related facilities. Reduced population growth alleviates congestion, improves traffic flow, and enhances transportation efficiency.

Slower population growth paves the way for a more strategic approach to housing planning and construction, ensuring a sufficient supply of housing to meet residents' needs. This results in better access to affordable housing, reduced housing shortages, and improved living conditions for all. Participating in voluntary abstinence and celibacy as well as population growth reduction programs are not just a personal choice for personal health or reduction in crime, but a ministry to save our planet and sustain our future. Additionally, a voluntarily controlled population growth rate enables better provision and management of sanitation and utility services. It facilitates the development of adequate infrastructure for clean water supply, wastewater treatment, and waste management. Consequently, this leads to improved public health, reduced environmental pollution, and overall better sanitation conditions in urban areas.

With a reduced rate of population growth, it becomes possible to plan and distribute public services and facilities such as schools, healthcare centers, parks, and community centers effectively. This ensures that everyone has equal access to essential public services, ultimately improving their quality of life and well-being.

Impact of Reduced Population Growth on Healthcare

A lower population growth rate can also positively impact healthcare systems, resulting in better access, reduced waiting times, and improved quality of care. Therefore, voluntary controlled population growth participation is achieved not through eugenics, government mandates, etc., but through public policy campaigns, incentives, and tax breaks to encourage and reward those who delay pregnancy, adopt children rather than birth their own, or just use self-control measures such as celibacy or abstinence can significantly contribute to the betterment of healthcare.

By reducing the population growth rate, healthcare systems become more efficient in providing services to everyone, leading to a lighter burden on healthcare facilities and increased availability of medical services like primary care, specialized treatments, and preventive care. As a result, everyone can receive prompt and appropriate healthcare whenever needed.

A lower population growth rate means fewer patients in healthcare facilities, resulting in shorter waiting times for appointments, diagnostic tests, surgeries, and other medical procedures. This reduction in wait times allows for more efficient and effective healthcare delivery, improving patient experiences and outcomes.

Voluntary controlled population growth enables better allocation of resources within healthcare systems. It allows healthcare providers to distribute healthcare professionals, medical equipment, medications, and funding more effectively. This ensures that resources are not overwhelmed, leading to improved efficiency and quality of care.

With reduced strain on healthcare facilities and improved resource allocation, healthcare providers can focus on delivering high-quality care to patients.

They can dedicate more time and attention to patients, provide comprehensive treatments, and ensure continuity of care. This contributes to better health outcomes and overall well-being for everyone.

Voluntary controlled population growth participation enables a targeted approach to preventive healthcare and public health initiatives. Healthcare systems can allocate resources to public health education, disease prevention programs, and early detection and intervention measures. This promotes population-wide health and helps reduce the burden of preventable diseases. By managing population growth and ensuring that healthcare systems can meet the needs of the population, everyone can experience improved access, shorter wait times, and better quality of care. This leads to better health outcomes, increased satisfaction with healthcare services, and overall enhanced well-being for Gen Xers and Millennials and communities.

Impact of Reduced Population Growth on Education

Controlling population growth can indeed result in improved educational opportunities for all. With the eventual reduction in the number of students in each classroom, educational institutions can offer more personalized attention to each student. This allows teachers to dedicate more time and resources to address the specific needs of students, creating a more tailored learning experience. Smaller class sizes facilitate better interaction between students and teachers, enhancing engagement and academic support, ultimately leading to better educational outcomes. Voluntary controlled population growth also enables educational institutions to allocate resources more effectively.

With a lower student population, educational facilities can provide the necessary resources, materials, and facilities, such as textbooks, technology, and extracurricular programs. This comprehensive approach helps students receive a well-rounded education. Additionally, a lower population growth rate creates a more suitable teaching and learning environment. Reduced overcrowding in schools fosters a calm and focused atmosphere, promoting student concentration and active participation. This contributes to a positive classroom environment that supports effective teaching and learning. Moreover, with a lower student-to-teacher ratio, teachers can customize their instruction to meet the unique needs and learning styles of all.

This personalized approach enables educators to offer targeted support, address learning gaps, and nurture the strengths and talents of each student, fostering an inclusive and supportive educational environment. Improved educational opportunities resulting from Voluntary controlled population growth can lead to better prospects for us in the future. Access to quality education equips students with essential knowledge, skills, and critical thinking abilities for personal development and success in various aspects

of life. It enhances their employability, career prospects, and overall socio-economic opportunities.

Impact of Reduced Population Growth on the Environment

Voluntary controlled population growth also plays a crucial role in alleviating environmental pressures. It promotes sustainability and reduces strain on ecosystems. With fewer people, the demand for natural resources, such as water, energy, and raw materials, decreases. This reduction in resource consumption helps conserve valuable resources and relieve strain on ecosystems. It enables a more sustainable use of resources and contributes to their long-term availability.

Voluntary controlled population growth encourages a shift towards sustainable consumption and production patterns. With a smaller population, there is less pressure on industries to overproduce goods and services. This can lead to more environmentally friendly practices, such as waste reduction, promoting recycling, and adopting cleaner production technologies.

Reducing our carbon footprint and preserving biodiversity can be achieved through voluntary participation in controlled population growth rate programs. By having fewer people, we can decrease energy consumption, transportation demands, and carbon-intensive activities, ultimately helping us reach emission reduction targets and create a more sustainable and climate-friendly future.

Additionally, lower population growth and reduced population concentrations can be achieved through an incentivized voluntary participation program, city move-out or move to the country programs which make living outside the city affordable, while at the same time maintaining practices to prevent encroachment on natural habitats and ecosystems, preserving biodiversity and safeguarding vulnerable species and ecosystems from human-induced pressures. Ultimately, non-government-mandated community-based voluntary participation in controlled incentivized population growth programs promotes ecological balance and ensures the long-term health and diversity of our natural environment.

Moreover, voluntary community-based controlled population growth promotes a strong sense of environmental responsibility and empowers communities to engage actively in environmental initiatives. When people free up energy that otherwise might go into sexual relationships or procreating, they unleash time and energy to focus on personal development or community improvements.

With a smaller population concentrations, there is a greater potential for community participation in conservation efforts, sustainable land use planning, and the protection of natural areas. This fosters a more sustainable and harmonious relationship with the environment. By effectively managing population growth and reducing strain on city resources, ecosystems, and natural resources, we enable sustainable practices, reduce carbon emissions, and contribute to the preservation of biodiversity and ecological balance. Some of these programs would require the development of high speed rail systems to make it practical for those who choose country living yet work in the city.

Ultimately, voluntary controlled population growth paves the way for a sustainable future and cultivates an environmentally conscious society. When we prioritize non-mandated population management, societies can strive towards achieving a balanced and sustainable future. However, it is crucial to approach population control ethically, respecting everyone's reproductive rights and considering spiritual, cultural, social, and economic factors. A comprehensive approach to population control includes education, access to family planning resources, empowerment of women, and sustainable development strategies. The author of this work makes clear that he strongly supports efforts that involve abstinence, celibacy, and pregnancy prevention methods rather than pregnancy termination efforts, which violate the rights of the unborn, who have a right to be born.

Chapter 4:
The Social Impact of Celibacy and Abstinence

Choosing celibacy and abstinence allows us to shift our focus towards personal growth, emotional well-being, and the development of strong, meaningful relationships outside of sexual involvement. By abstaining from sexual relationships, we have the opportunity to prioritize our own development. Without the distractions and time commitments of sexual interactions, we can dedicate more time and energy to self-reflection, introspection, and pursuing personal goals. This can involve exploring hobbies, acquiring new skills, pursuing passions, and working towards personal aspirations. Voluntary non-mandated celibacy and abstinence facilitate self-discovery, self-improvement, and a deeper understanding of oneself.

Abstaining from sexual activities also enables us to cultivate a healthier relationship with their emotions and sexuality.

It involves developing emotional intelligence, self-awareness, and self-control. It allows us to establish a strong sense of self-worth and confidence, independent of their sexual experiences.

Celibacy and abstinence promote emotional stability, inner peace, and a greater sense of contentment. By redirecting our energy away from sexual involvement, we can focus on building deep, meaningful connections with others based on shared values, emotional intimacy, and mutual respect. This fosters the cultivation of strong friendships, emotional support networks, and non-sexual romantic relationships. By nurturing these relationships, we can experience companionship, love, and a sense of belonging without relying on sexual interactions.

Moreover, celibacy and abstinence provide an opportunity to explore and cultivate different forms of intimacy beyond sexuality. This includes emotional intimacy, intellectual connection, and spiritual bonding. By redirecting our focus towards these aspects, we can develop rich and fulfilling relationships that go beyond physical attraction. Embracing celibacy and abstinence can align with personal values and priorities, allowing us to live in accordance with our beliefs, whether influenced by cultural, religious, or personal convictions. This alignment promotes a sense of integrity, authenticity, and personal fulfillment. By embracing celibacy and abstinence, we can prioritize personal growth, enhance emotional well-being, and build deep and meaningful connections with others. It offers an alternative path to self-discovery, personal satisfaction, and the cultivation of fulfilling relationships beyond the realm of sexual involvement.

Adopting celibacy and abstinence can contribute to cultivating a culture that values emotional intelligence, respect, and deeper connections based on shared values and mutual understanding. Celibacy and abstinence encourage us to develop emotional intelligence by focusing on self-awareness, empathy, and effective communication. By placing greater emphasis on emotional connection and understanding, we can nurture stronger emotional intelligence skills, leading to more satisfying and meaningful relationships. This promotes a culture where emotional intelligence is highly regarded and nurtured. By embracing celibacy and abstinence, we prioritize respect in our relationships, including respect for personal boundaries, consent, and individual autonomy. Building a culture of respect fosters healthier and more equitable relationships where all parties feel valued, heard, and understood. It encourages open communication, mutual support, and empathy.

Intellectual Conversations

The exploration of deeper intellectual conversations

fosters a culture where communication is valued, vulnerability is embraced, and deeper connections are sought after. When we engage in discussions that transcend superficial topics, they create an environment that encourages open and meaningful communication. By actively listening to one another, expressing thoughts and ideas, and engaging in thoughtful dialogue, we foster an atmosphere where communication is given importance and respected.

In these intellectual conversations, we can delve into topics that require vulnerability. Sharing personal experiences, perspectives, and opinions on deeper matters can be a vulnerable act; however, in an environment that values intellectual conversations, we can feel more comfortable expressing our thoughts and emotions. This willingness to be vulnerable fosters trust, authenticity, and deeper connections as we share our genuine selves and engage in honest and meaningful interactions.

Furthermore, the pursuit of deeper intellectual connections signifies a yearning for more profound relationships. By engaging in conversations that delve into ideas and stimulate the mind, we demonstrate a willingness to surpass superficial interactions characterized by our predecessors. We can seek connections built on shared values, intellectual curiosity, and a mutual appreciation for intellectual growth. This pursuit of deeper connections enables us to form relationships that transcend mere physical attraction, fostering a sense of satisfaction and contentment in our interactions. The culture of valuing communication, embracing vulnerability, and seeking deeper connections nurtured by these intellectual conversations has wide-ranging effects on our four generations (Boomers, X'rs, Y'rs, Millennials, and Alpha).

At this interpersonal level, by participating in these conversations, we proceed toward personal growth and a sense of inner and interpersonal fulfillment. We can expand our knowledge, broaden our perspectives, and deepen our understanding of each other. Through meaningful exchanges, we can challenge our own assumptions, learn from different viewpoints, and develop a more comprehensive worldview. These experiences contribute to personal development and the cultivation of intellectual curiosity.

On a societal level, a culture that values communication, embraces vulnerability, and seeks deeper connections, fosters a more empathetic and understanding society. Intellectual conversations promote dialogue, encourage the exploration of diverse perspectives, and facilitate the resolution of conflicts through thoughtful discussion. They create a space where we can appreciate and respect differences while finding common ground and shared understanding. This, in turn, contributes to the development of a more inclusive and cohesive society. It's important to note this must be an organic and voluntary process not spearheaded by government or special interests.

Impact of Celibacy and Abstinence on Social Connection

Choosing celibacy or abstinence opens up the door

for us to form connections beyond purely sexual encounters. By refraining from engaging in sexual activity, we can partake in various activities together more consistently, explore shared hobbies, discover new places, or collaborate on meaningful projects and see them through without sexual entanglements that get in the way. These shared experiences foster a sense of connection, bonding, and understanding between us, establishing a strong foundation for more profound and meaningful relationships on a wider scale.

Engaging in activities together enables us to create richer shared memories and nurture a deeper sense of camaraderie beyond the sexual encounter. Whether it involves embarking on adventures, attending events, or simply enjoying quality time, these experiences generate a bond rooted in shared pleasure and mutual interests. By immersing ourselves in activities that extend beyond the realm of sex, we have the opportunity to build connections that are not solely centered around physical intimacy.

Shared hobbies also serve as avenues for connection

and personal growth. Pursuing common interests such as sports, art, music, or other recreational activities allows us to explore our passions alongside like-minded others. This shared pursuit of personal fulfillment and enjoyment establishes common ground and strengthens the bonds between individuals, facilitating the development of deeper connections based on shared experiences and a genuine appreciation for each other's interests.

Exploring new environments together through traveling, discovering new cultures, or embarking on adventures can foster a sense of shared discovery and excitement, connecting us beyond sexual encounters; or by making the relationship non-sexual for a period, we can develop a foundation of friendship, trust, and honesty that when mutually agreed upon, will enhance the sexual experience beyond a casual encounter [monogamy or marriage] with an experience beyond measure. These experiences provide an opportunity to gain a deeper understanding of one another and forge a connection that extends beyond physical attraction. Moreover, engaging in these activities encourages teamwork, communication, and cooperation, all of which contribute to the development of stronger relationships.

Similarly, participating in meaningful projects such as volunteering, activism, or community initiatives allows us to connect on a deeper level. Collaborating towards a common goal enables us to bond over shared values and a sense of purpose. This fosters unity, compassion, and empathy, bringing us closer together and cultivating a sense of collective responsibility. By focusing on shared experiences and activities, celibacy and abstinence create opportunities for us to form connections that are based on more than just sexual encounters.

Chapter 5:
Economic Impact of Celibacy and Abstinence

When we choose celibacy or practice abstinence, we actively take measures to prevent unintended pregnancies. By abstaining from sexual activity, the risk of pregnancy significantly decreases. This reduction in unplanned pregnancies can relieve the burden on public resources allocated to supporting families facing financial difficulties. With fewer unplanned pregnancies, there may be a decrease in the number of families in need of welfare programs. This reduced demand allows for a more focused and sustainable approach to social support. The limited resources available for welfare programs can be directed towards those who are most in need, ensuring that the support reaches those who require it the most.

Moreover, the decrease in unplanned pregnancies resulting from celibacy and abstinence can also have positive implications for healthcare services related to prenatal care and childbirth. When pregnancies are planned, we have the opportunity to seek appropriate prenatal care, reducing the risks associated with inadequate or delayed healthcare. This can lead to improved health outcomes for both the mother and the child.

However, it is important to note that celibacy and abstinence should be presented as options among a range of choices. The focus should be on providing everyone with comprehensive education that includes information about contraception, safe sex practices, and the importance of family planning that does not involve terminating pregnancies out of inconvenience. This empowers us to make decisions that align with our values and circumstances while reducing the risk of unplanned pregnancies.

Unplanned pregnancies necessitate access to prenatal care and healthcare services related to childbirth. With a lower number of unplanned pregnancies, there is less strain on healthcare systems, allowing for the more effective utilization of healthcare resources. This can result in better access, shorter waiting times, and improved quality of care for anyone in need of reproductive healthcare services.

Planned pregnancies have been shown to result in better prenatal care and health outcomes compared to unplanned pregnancies. Encouraging celibacy and abstinence enables us to have greater control over our reproductive choices, allowing us to plan pregnancies when we are physically, emotionally, and financially prepared. This, in turn, can lead to healthier pregnancies, fewer complications, and improved health outcomes for both mothers and children.

In conclusion, a decrease in the demand for public resources related to unplanned pregnancies also enables more efficient allocation of resources in other crucial areas, such as education, infrastructure, and public services. This reallocation of funds and capacity allows for addressing other societal needs and priorities, contributing to overall social and economic development. By reducing unplanned pregnancies through celibacy and abstinence, public resources can be better targeted and utilized beyond welfare programs and reproductive healthcare services. This strategic allocation of resources supports broader societal needs and enhances the overall well-being of all.

Chapter 6:
Global Impact

Implementing celibacy and abstinence as measures for population control can make a significant contribution to addressing environmental challenges. By reducing resource consumption, carbon emissions, and ecological strain, these practices can help mitigate the impact on the planet. Curbing population growth through celibacy and abstinence decreases the demand for resources such as food, water, energy, and raw materials. This reduction in resource consumption not only eases the pressure on ecosystems but also promotes a more sustainable use of natural resources. By choosing celibacy and abstinence, we have the power to alleviate strain on the environment and foster long-term sustainability. I believe the impact of choosing this path over others mentioned can be experienced immediately, locally, and globally within our lifetimes.

One of the primary environmental benefits of population control through celibacy and abstinence lies in reduced demand for food. As the global population continues to grow, so does the need for food. This high demand puts immense pressure on agricultural systems, leading to deforestation, habitat destruction, and excessive use of water and fertilizers. However, by practicing celibacy or abstinence, we can contribute to slowing down population growth, thereby reducing the strain on food production systems and supporting more sustainable agricultural practices. It must be noted for those who choose celibacy and abstinence in service to their community or country should be provided with opportunities to redirect their reproductive energy into meaningful self development efforts, incentives, and rewards for their sacrifice.

Furthermore, reduced population growth resulting from celibacy and abstinence also plays a crucial role in decreasing the demand for water resources. Water scarcity remains a pressing environmental concern in many regions worldwide. However, by having fewer people, the strain on freshwater sources decreases, preserving this valuable resource. This reduction in demand allows for better water management, reduced pollution, and improved ecosystem health.

We might even consider funding an experimental non-religious living communities composed of those individuals or couples who choose abstinence in their relationship, between relationships, celibacy, monogamy, or marriage as a way of life in order to devote themselves to some endeavor be practical or spiritual. These would be people who's individual or group pursuit is to produce something of benefit to society whether it be in the arts, sciences, policy, etc. Entrance into or exit from this community voluntary without stigma or judgement.

Moreover, population control through celibacy and abstinence leads to reduced energy consumption and carbon emissions. A smaller population translates to lower energy demands for residential, commercial, and transportation purposes. Consequently, there is a decreased reliance on fossil fuels, resulting in decreased greenhouse gas emissions and a more sustainable energy future. By curbing population growth, we can actively contribute to mitigating positive climate change and addressing the environmental impact associated with energy production and consumption.

Additionally, population control through celibacy and abstinence can alleviate the strain on ecosystems caused by human activities, such as habitat destruction and deforestation. As the population grows at a slower rate, there is less pressure to convert natural areas into urban and agricultural landscapes. This allows for the preservation and restoration of ecosystems, protection of biodiversity, and maintenance of vital ecological services.

Voluntary controlled population growth through celibacy and abstinence can help preserve ecological balance by reducing habitat destruction and fragmentation. It minimizes encroachment on natural habitats, thus protecting biodiversity and wildlife populations. Preserving ecological balance is crucial for maintaining healthy ecosystems and safeguarding the planet's natural resources. By adopting celibacy and abstinence, we can embrace more sustainable lifestyles, prioritizing simplicity, conscious consumption, and eco-friendly practices. This can include reduced waste generation, energy conservation, and a focus on renewable resources. Such sustainable lifestyles contribute to environmental preservation and alleviate the ecological strain caused by human activities.

Population control through celibacy and abstinence can promote environmental education and advocacy, fostering our awareness of the environmental challenges we face and encouraging action to protect and restore our planet. It cultivates a culture of environmental stewardship and engagement in sustainable activities. By managing population growth through celibacy and abstinence, we can contribute to mitigating environmental challenges, reducing resource consumption, lowering carbon emissions, and preserving ecological balance. However, I will reiterate that it is crucial to approach population control ethically, respecting reproductive rights and considering broader socio-economic factors. Additionally, comprehensive strategies addressing sustainable development, conservation practices, and responsible resource management are essential for long-term environmental sustainability.

Addressing Overpopulation

Population control through celibacy and abstinence can address overpopulation issues in regions with limited resources, helping achieve a more sustainable balance between human needs and the environment. In such regions, high population growth rates can deplete resources and create scarcity. By practicing celibacy and abstinence, we can alleviate strain on limited resources such as water, land, and food, enabling more sustainable utilization and ensuring their availability for present and future generations.

Overpopulation, in addition to environmental degradation, including deforestation, often leads to habitat loss and pollution. By controlling population growth through celibacy and abstinence, pressure on natural ecosystems is reduced, lowering the risk of environmental damage. This promotes the preservation of ecosystems, biodiversity, and overall environmental health. Achieving a sustainable balance between human needs and the environment requires careful resource and ecosystem management, where population control plays a vital role. Embracing celibacy and abstinence allow us to contribute to sustainable development practices and maintain a healthy equilibrium.

Overpopulation can strain socio-economic systems, leading to increased poverty, unemployment, and social inequality. However, managing population growth through celibacy and abstinence can help regions achieve a more stable socio-economic environment. A balanced population size allows for better resource distribution, improved access to healthcare and education, and reduced socio-economic disparities. Population control through celibacy and abstinence offers numerous socio-economic benefits, fostering a more equitable and sustainable society.

When a region experiences overpopulation, resources can become scarce and insufficient to meet the growing population's needs. This scarcity can result in increased poverty and unemployment rates as limited resources are stretched thin. By practicing celibacy or choosing abstinence, we can managing population growth and alleviating strain on socio-economic systems. This balanced approach enables a more equitable distribution of resources, ensuring access to basic necessities such as food, housing, and employment opportunities.

Moreover, managed population growth resulting from celibacy and abstinence allows regions to allocate resources more effectively for healthcare and education. With a smaller population, there is a reduced burden on healthcare systems, leading to improved access to quality healthcare services. Adequate healthcare provision contributes to better health outcomes, reduced healthcare costs, and an overall healthier population.

Similarly, in the realm of education, a balanced population size allows for more effective education systems, ensuring improved access to quality education for everyone. This contributes to enhanced human capital development and increased opportunities for social and economic mobility.

Addressing Social Inequality

Addressing social inequality can also be achieved by promoting celibacy and abstinence as measures to reduce population growth. Overpopulation exacerbates socioeconomic disparities as resources become concentrated in specific areas or among certain groups. By managing population growth, regions can work towards a more equitable society where we have equal opportunities for advancement and prosperity. A more balanced population size allows for a more even distribution of resources and reduces the disparities that often arise in overpopulated areas.

Managing population growth through celibacy and abstinence provides numerous socio-economic benefits. By curbing overpopulation, regions can achieve a more stable socio-economic environment. This approach promotes better resource distribution, improved access to healthcare and education, and reduced socio-economic disparities. By practicing celibacy or choosing abstinence, we contribute to creating a more equitable and sustainable society where socio-economic opportunities are more widely accessible and socio-economic disparities are reduced.

Indeed, overpopulation significantly impacts our quality of life, resulting in challenges related to access to basic amenities, overcrowding, and social issues. However, by promoting population control, particularly in regions facing limited resources, we can experience a better quality of life. This includes improved access to healthcare, education, and a healthier environment.

Chapter 7:
The Historical Origins of Celibacy and Abstinence

Throughout history, numerous influential figures and movements have stressed the importance of celibacy and abstinence as a way of life. These individuals and groups have advocated for the virtues of abstinence for religious, spiritual, philosophical, or personal reasons. Their promotion of celibacy and abstinence has had a profound influence on society, shaping cultural, religious, and philosophical perspectives. By examining some prominent figures and movements that have emphasized celibacy and abstinence, we gain insight into the diverse historical contexts and motivations behind these practices.

One notable example is the ancient Greek philosopher Socrates, who advocated for a life of sexual abstinence as a means to concentrate on intellectual pursuits and the pursuit of wisdom. Socrates believed that sexual desires and distractions could hinder the search for truth and the development of one's intellectual capacities. His teachings influenced many followers and shaped the philosophical discussions of his time.

In the realm of religion, figures such as Saint Anthony of Egypt and Saint Thérèse of Lisieux are well-known for their commitment to celibacy and abstinence. Saint Anthony, considered the founder of Christian monasticism, lived a life of extreme asceticism, renouncing worldly pleasures and embracing celibacy to dedicate himself entirely to his spiritual journey. Saint Thérèse, a French Carmelite nun, followed a similar path, choosing celibacy as a means to fully devote herself to prayer, contemplation, and service to others.

In more recent history, the counter-cultural movements of the 1960s and 1970s brought attention to celibacy and abstinence as a way to challenge societal norms and seek spiritual or personal liberation. The sexual revolution and associated movements, such as the hippie counterculture, emphasized sexual freedom and exploration. However, there were individuals and groups within these movements who embraced celibacy and abstinence as a rejection of mainstream culture and as a way to focus on inner transformation and spiritual growth.

Religious and spiritual communities worldwide have also placed a strong emphasis on celibacy and abstinence. In traditions such as Buddhism, Jainism, and certain sects of Hinduism, celibacy is considered a noble and virtuous path. Monks, nuns, and spiritual practitioners within these traditions commit themselves to a life of celibacy as part of their spiritual practice, seeking liberation, enlightenment, or a deeper connection with the divine.

These examples highlight the wide range of historical figures and movements that have emphasized celibacy and abstinence. From philosophers to religious leaders, counter-cultural movements to spiritual communities, the motivations for embracing celibacy and abstinence have been diverse and deeply rooted in personal beliefs, values, and cultural contexts.

The Sexual Revolution

The sexual revolution and its related movements, such as the hippie counterculture, caused significant shifts in attitudes towards sexuality, relationships, and personal freedom. These movements brought both newfound openness and exploration, as well as various impacts and costs in healthcare, social, economic, spiritual, and cultural aspects.

Looking at healthcare, the sexual revolution and the widespread acceptance of sexual freedom had implications for public health. The increase in sexual activity and multiple partners led to a higher risk of sexually transmitted infections (STIs) and unintended pregnancies. Insufficient knowledge about safe sex practices and contraception during this time contributed to the spread of STIs and the need for reproductive healthcare services. Furthermore, the sexual revolution challenged traditional norms and sparked debates around reproductive rights, contraception, and abortion, which remain significant social and healthcare topics. The sexual revolution may, in part or in whole, be directly responsible for the break of the nuclear family and the deterioration of traditional family values.

On a social level, the sexual revolution questioned established social and cultural norms surrounding sexuality and relationships. It ignited discussions and debates about gender roles, sexual orientation, and the concept of consent. The emphasis on sexual freedom and exploration resulted in changes in societal attitudes towards premarital sex, cohabitation, and non-traditional relationships. While these changes brought increased acceptance and inclusivity, they also contributed to divisions in society and moral debates concerning the importance of marriage and family values.

Economically, the sexual revolution had implications for industries associated with sexuality and relationships. For instance, the pornography industry experienced growth alongside the increased acceptance of sexual expression. However, this industry, as well as the broader commercialization of sex, raised concerns about objectification, exploitation, and their impact on Boomer, Gen Xers, Gen Y, Millennial, and now Gen Alpha relationships today. The commodification of sexuality and the emphasis on physical appearance also fueled consumerism and societal pressures related to body image and self-worth.

From a spiritual perspective, the sexual revolution challenged traditional religious teachings and practices regarding sexuality and morality. The emphasis on personal freedom and exploration clashed with conservative religious views on premarital sex, homosexuality, and contraception. This led to tensions and debates within religious communities and created divisions among those adhering to different religious or spiritual beliefs.

Culturally, the sexual revolution brought about changes in cultural norms and popular culture. It influenced the depiction of sexuality in music, literature, film, and art and opened up discussions about previously taboo subjects. While this cultural shift contributed to greater artistic expression and freedom of speech, it also sparked debates about the impact of explicit content on societal values, particularly among younger audiences.

In conclusion, the sexual revolution and its associated movements had complex impacts and consequences in healthcare, social, economic, spiritual, and cultural realms. While they brought about greater openness and exploration, they also raised public health costs, concerns about public health, challenged social norms, ignited moral debates, influenced economic industries, affected population growth, created conditions which fostered unwanted pregnancies, exacerbated conditions which increased poverty, crime, resource strain, and generated tensions within religious communities. Understanding and navigating the consequences of these movements continue to shape ongoing discussions and debates in various aspects of society. It is clear that we must reverse the impact of the sexual revolution.

Reversing the Impact of the Sexual Revolution

Promoting celibacy and abstinence alone would not be enough to completely undo the impact of the sexual revolution. The sexual revolution brought about significant changes in attitudes, behaviors, and societal norms surrounding sexuality and relationships. These effects are deeply ingrained in the cultural and social perspectives of subsequent generations and cannot be easily reversed by advocating celibacy and abstinence.

While celibacy and abstinence can be personal choices made for various reasons, such as religious beliefs, personal values, or health considerations, advocating for them on a large scale would not erase the changes brought about by the sexual revolution. The sexual revolution challenged traditional norms and led to greater acceptance of sexual freedom, exploration, and diverse forms of relationships. It sparked discussions about consent, gender equality, and sexual orientation. These shifts in societal attitudes have influenced laws, policies, and cultural representations related to sexuality and relationships.

To reverse the impact of the sexual revolution, broader changes in attitudes, education, and cultural narratives are necessary. This involves promoting comprehensive sexual education that emphasizes informed decision-making, consent, safe sex practices, and healthy relationships. It requires addressing the underlying factors that contribute to issues like sexual violence, gender inequality, and unhealthy relationship dynamics.

Reestablishing a balanced approach to sexuality and relationships means fostering a culture that values consent, open communication, mutual respect, and

personal agency. It requires promoting healthy relationships, addressing social inequalities, and dismantling harmful gender norms. All of this can be accom-
plished if our society as a whole paused the sexual
revolution drumbeat that has seduced us all to redirect our sexual energy toward personal growth, improved interpersonal communication, and community health and well-being.

While celibacy and abstinence are valid choices for
us, it is important to recognize that everyone has diverse experiences, beliefs, and desires related to their
sexuality, so none of this should be forced. Emphasizing the importance of choice, consent, and personal
well-being is crucial in supporting our' autonomy
and fostering a culture of sexual empowerment and
healthy relationships.

In conclusion, the impact of the sexual revolution
cannot be completely reversed through the widespread adoption of celibacy and abstinence alone. Re-
versing its impact requires comprehensive efforts
that involve education, cultural and spiritual shifts,

addressing social inequalities, and promoting healthy attitudes and behaviors related to sexuality and relationships. We have long passed the question of "Should we?" and are down the road toward "How long do we need to do this?"

Chapter 8:
Advantages of Celibacy and Abstinence

Choosing celibacy and abstinence offers immediate benefits for all of us. Firstly, abstaining from sexual activity provides a powerful method of protection against sexually transmitted infections (STIs). By avoiding intimate contact, we eliminate the risk of contracting or transmitting STIs, which can have significant health consequences. This short-term benefit promotes sexual health and reduces the need for medical interventions, treatments, and the potential emotional and physical toll that comes with dealing with STIs. Thereby decreasing our healthcare costs and avoiding infections that could go undiagnosed and lead to life-threatening illnesses.

In addition to physical health, celibacy and abstinence can contribute to emotional and mental well-being. Choosing to abstain from sexual relationships can provide us with a sense of control over their own bodies and lives. This sense of control can lead to reduced stress, anxiety, and emotional turmoil often associated with sexual relationships. By removing the pressures and complexities of sexual involvement, we may experience a greater sense of emotional stability, mental clarity, and overall well-being. This greater sense of emotional stability, mental clarity, and overall well-being can be harnessed and directed toward faster mastery of skills and quicker attainment of goals.

Moreover, one of the immediate benefits of celibacy and abstinence is the avoidance of unintended pregnancies. By abstaining from sexual activity, we may eliminate further risks of unintended pregnancies and the potential challenges and responsibilities associated with them. This benefit allows us to focus on our own personal goals, aspirations, and self-development without the added responsibilities and life-altering decisions that come with parenthood. The ability to pursue education, career advancement, and personal growth unhindered by the demands of parenthood can lead to a sense of freedom, empowerment, and self-fulfillment in the short term.

Furthermore, practicing celibacy and abstinence can cultivate self-discipline and self-control. By making a conscious choice to abstain from sexual activity, we may exercise control over our desires and develop a stronger sense of self-mastery. This practice of self-discipline can extend beyond the realm of sexuality and positively impact other areas of life that require discipline and self-control. It can strengthen will-power, enhance decision-making skills, and foster a greater sense of personal empowerment.

Short-Term and Long-Term Benefits of Celibacy and Abstinence

The short-term benefits of celibacy and abstinence can positively impact various aspects of our lives. From protecting against STIs and promoting sexual health to fostering emotional well-being and personal growth, the decision to practice celibacy and abstinence can lead to immediate advantages. These benefits include physical health, emotional stability, the avoidance of unintended pregnancies, and the cultivation of self-discipline and self-control. It is important to note that the benefits may vary for each, and the decision to practice celibacy and abstinence should align with personal beliefs, values, and circumstances.

In addition to the short-term benefits, celibacy and abstinence can bring about long-term advantages that positively impact mental and physical health, relationships, lifespan, and spiritual development. One of the long-term benefits of celibacy and abstinence is improved mental health. By abstaining from sexual relationships, we may experience reduced stress, anxiety, and emotional turmoil commonly associated with sexual dynamics. This can lead to improved mental well-being, increased emotional stability, and enhanced overall psychological health. The freedom from the complexities and challenges of sexual relationships can contribute to a greater sense of inner peace, contentment, and emotional resilience over time.

Health Benefits of Celibacy and Abstinence

Engaging in sexual activity carries certain health risks and consequences, and choosing celibacy and abstinence can help mitigate these risks. By refraining from sexual relationships, we can potentially reduce the transmission and acquisition of sexually transmitted infections (STIs). This includes common STIs such as chlamydia, gonorrhea, herpes, and HIV/AIDS. Avoiding exposure to these infections decreases the likelihood of long-term health complications associated with STIs, such as chronic infections, infertility, and increased vulnerability to other infections or diseases.

In addition to STIs, celibacy and abstinence can positively impact overall physical health. Sexual activity often involves physical exertion, which, pleasurable as this may be, can be demanding on the body if done immoderately, particularly as age, too much sex with too many sexual partners may engender poor outcomes, diminished health, etc. By choosing celibacy and abstinence from time to time, we can potentially decrease the risk of physical strain, injuries, and complications that may arise from excessive sexual activity. This promotes better physical well-being and a healthier body over the long term.

Furthermore, practicing celibacy and abstinence can lead to healthier reproductive health outcomes. By avoiding sexual relationships, we decrease the risk of certain reproductive health issues, such as cervical and prostate cancer, which have been linked to human papillomavirus (HPV) and Chlamydia sexually transmitted infections. These types of cancers can have serious health implications and may require invasive treatments, such as surgery, radiation, or chemotherapy. By opting for celibacy and abstinence, we can potentially decrease our vulnerability to these types of cancers and maintain better reproductive health.

It is important to note that while celibacy and abstinence can reduce the risk of certain reproductive health issues, they do not guarantee complete protection. Regular screenings, such as Pap tests for cervical cancer and prostate-specific antigen (PSA) tests for prostate cancer, remain important for early detection and effective management of these conditions. Additionally, other risk factors beyond sexual activity, such as genetics and lifestyle choices, can also influence the development of these cancers. Celibacy and abstinence contribute to a reduced risk of certain reproductive health issues such as cervical and prostate cancer.

Spiritual Benefits of Celibacy and Abstinence

Beyond the societal and health advantages, celibacy and abstinence also offer us the opportunity for spiritual growth and a deeper connection to their chosen spiritual path. Throughout various religious and spiritual traditions, celibacy has long been embraced as a form of spiritual devotion. By abstaining from sexual relationships, we can redirect our energy and focus toward spiritual pursuits and personal development. This intentional shift allows us to cultivate a stronger sense of spirituality, exploring our connection to higher ideals, inner peace, and a higher power.

For many practicing celibacy and abstinence, the absence of sexual relationships creates space for introspection, reflection, and contemplation. This inner journey can lead to a greater understanding of oneself, personal values, and the purpose of life. By redirecting our energy away from physical desires, we may find a sense of liberation and clarity that fosters spiritual growth and a deeper connection to our own spiritual beliefs and practices.

Moreover, celibacy and abstinence can facilitate the development of discipline, self-control, and mindfulness, which are fundamental aspects of many spiritual traditions. By consciously choosing to abstain from sexual activity, we exercise discipline over our desires and cultivate a heightened sense of self-mastery. This discipline can extend beyond sexuality and positively influence other areas of life, including the cultivation of spiritual practices such as meditation, prayer, and self-reflection.

Additionally, celibacy and abstinence provide us with an opportunity to establish a deeper connection with our chosen spiritual community. Embracing the values and practices of celibacy often leads us to become part of a larger community that shares similar beliefs and aspirations. This sense of belonging and shared commitment to spiritual growth can provide a support system and nourish one's spiritual journey, fostering a sense of camaraderie and collective purpose.

Furthermore, practicing celibacy and abstinence can create an environment that fosters heightened sensitivity and awareness. By redirecting focus away from physical desires, we may become more attuned to our own spiritual experiences, subtle energies, and the spiritual dimensions of life. This increased sensitivity can deepen our connection to the divine, facilitate spiritual insights, and enhance their overall spiritual journey.

Chapter 9:
The Connection Between Self-control and Societal Well-being

Rome, the Maya, Easter Island, the Anasazi, and Spartan Civilization

Societies throughout history have faced decline or collapse due to factors like over-consumption, resource depletion, and environmental degradation. These factors are often tied to a lack of self-control and restraint. By studying past instances of societal decline, we can understand the importance of self-control and restraint in shaping societies. A prime example of decline caused by a lack of self-control is the fall of the Roman Empire. The empire's excessive lifestyle and unrestrained use of resources led to environmental degradation and resource scarcity.

Moreover, political corruption and instability further weakened the empire, eventually leading to its downfall.

The decline of the Roman Empire was a result of various factors, including moral decay, excessive indulgence in luxuries, and a decline in discipline and moderation, alongside other challenges on political, economic, and military fronts. In his book, "The History of the Decline and Fall of the Roman Empire," Edward Gibbon identifies political corruption, instability, economic troubles, over-reliance on slave labor, military overspending, over-expansion, and invasion by barbarian tribes as reasons for the empire's downfall. It seems that the absence of self-control and self-restraint played a significant role in each of these identified reasons. While Gibbon did not explicitly discuss celibacy and abstinence as preventive measures against the decline of the empire, he did emphasize the importance of moral decay and a decline in civic virtue. It is possible that he may have viewed practices such as celibacy and abstinence as contributing to the maintenance of moral standards, although further evidence is needed to confirm this.

Indeed, the fall of the Mayan civilization serves as an example of the consequences of population growth, resource depletion, and the inability to effectively address these challenges. The Maya, who were organized in city-states, experienced rapid population growth in certain areas, which put substantial pressure on the available resources. To sustain a large population for an extended period, the Maya developed advanced agricultural techniques like terracing, irrigation systems, and the cultivation of crops like maize. However, as the population continued to increase, the demands on land and resources grew, leading to environmental degradation and resource depletion.

The unsustainable agricultural practices, along with deforestation, soil erosion, and the depletion of fertile land, resulted in a decline in agricultural productivity. This decline, combined with social issues, ultimately led to the downfall of the Mayan civilization and political instability caused by resource scarcity, contributed to the collapse of some Mayan city-states and the overall decline of the civilization. The decline of the Mayan civilization was largely attributed to their failure to effectively manage population growth, resource consumption, and environmental sustainability. This strain on resources, combined with political and social difficulties, weakened the civilization's resilience and eventually led to the fragmentation and abandonment of major urban centers. Certainly, the practice of self-control and self-restraint, by-products of the regular practice of abstinence and celibacy, would have had a positive impact on the survival of their civilization other things considered.

The examples of Easter Island and the Mayan civilization should serve as reminders of the crucial role played by self-control, responsible resource management, and sustainable practices in ensuring the long-term viability and resilience of societies. They emphasize the importance of balancing population growth with resource availability, environmental preservation, and societal stability to avoid the dangers of overconsumption and environmental degradation. The story of Easter Island acts as a cautionary tale, illustrating the severe consequences that can arise from the absence of self-control and excessive consumption. The Rapa Nui civilization, which inhabited Easter Island, faced significant challenges due to their unsustainable resource management practices.

As the population of Easter Island grew, the demand for resources increased. The Rapa Nui heavily relied on the island's forests for various purposes, such as building massive stone statues called moai. However, their excessive use of natural resources resulted in widespread deforestation. This had negative consequences for the island's ecosystem, including soil erosion, loss of biodiversity, and a decline in available resources.

The ecological imbalance caused by the over-exploitation of resources, combined with internal conflicts and scarcity, contributed to the decline of Rapa Nui society. The depletion of resources made it difficult for the civilization to sustain itself, leading to a collapse of their social structures.

The Easter Island example emphasizes the importance of self-control and responsible resource management for long-term sustainability. It demonstrates the negative effects that can occur when consumption is unchecked, and resource utilization lacks restraint. The cautionary tale of Easter Island serves as a reminder of the need for sustainable practices and careful stewardship of our natural environment to prevent the decline and potential collapse of societies.

The Anasazi civilization, also known as the Ancestral Puebloans, encountered difficulties due to overpopulation, resource depletion, and environmental change, which ultimately led to their downfall. The Anasazi developed advanced agricultural techniques, such as constructing intricate irrigation systems and cultivating maize (corn), which allowed them to sustain a relatively large population in their dry surroundings.

However, as time went on, the Anasazi population grew, placing greater strain on the available resources. Their agricultural practices, combined with a shifting climate and environmental factors, resulted in the depletion of vital resources like water and wood. The mounting pressure on these resources, along with extended periods of drought and other environmental challenges, made it increasingly challenging for the Anasazi to maintain their agricultural productivity and support their population.

The inability to effectively manage population growth and adapt to changing environmental conditions significantly contributed to the decline of the Anasazi civilization. As resources became scarce, competition for essential goods intensified, leading to social unrest and conflicts within the community. These factors, combined with the impact of environmental change, ultimately led to the abandonment of numerous Anasazi settlements and the decline of their civilization.

It should be noted that the decline of the Anasazi civilization was a complex process affected by various factors, including how resources were managed, climate change, societal dynamics, and external pressures. Although overpopulation and depletion of resources played a significant role, they were just part of a larger set of challenges that impacted the sustainability and resilience of Anasazi society.

In contrast, ancient Sparta stands as a notable example of a society that highly valued self-control and discipline, distinguishing it from civilizations like Rome, the Maya, Easter Island, and the Anasazi. The city-state of Sparta placed great importance on adhering to strict codes of conduct and practicing self-discipline in different aspects of life, particularly in military training and daily routines. This unwavering commitment to self-control played a crucial role in shaping the fate of Spartan society.

The Spartans fostered a culture of discipline from an early age, instilling self-control as a fundamental virtue. Their military training, known as the agoge, aimed to shape individuals with exceptional physical and mental strength. Through demanding physical exercises, strict discipline, and rigorous social norms, the Spartans created a formidable military force renowned for their endurance, bravery, and unwavering loyalty.

The military prowess of the Spartans was greatly attributed to their focus on self-control, which also played a crucial role in maintaining stability within their society. By adhering to strict codes of conduct and practicing social discipline, the citizens of Sparta fostered a sense of order, unity, and purpose. This disciplined approach enabled Sparta to withstand internal conflicts and external threats and retain political stability over a long period of time.

The case of ancient Sparta, with its emphasis on self-control, highlights the significant impact this virtue has on shaping the destiny of historical societies. It demonstrates how self-control can influence not only military strength but also societal stability and the overall trajectory of civilizations throughout history.

These examples serve as a powerful reminder of the profound significance of self-control, or the lack thereof, in determining the fate of historical societies. They emphasize the enduring value of cultivating self-discipline, restraint, and adherence to codes of conduct, as these qualities can profoundly shape the success, resilience, and longevity of civilizations.

Chinese Civilization

Let's examine one of the oldest civilizations that dates back to ancient times. Ancient China has a history of 5,000 years and is widely regarded as one of the most continuously enduring civilizations in the present era. It's important to acknowledge that the rise and fall of civilizations are influenced by various factors, with self-control being just one aspect among many that contribute to their destiny. Self-control has played a significant role in the longevity of Chinese civilization. Throughout its extensive history, self-control has been emphasized as a fundamental virtue in Chinese culture and has contributed to the stability and resilience of their civilization. One of the key factors contributing to the longevity of Chinese civilization is the emphasis on self-control.

Chinese philosophical systems such as Confucianism, Taoism, and Buddhism have placed great importance on the cultivation of self-control as a means to achieve personal and societal harmony. These teachings advocate for the practice of self-discipline, restraint, and the development of virtuous behavior. By adhering to these principles, individuals within their culture contribute to the preservation of social order, ethical standards, and cultural continuity over the course of centuries. Self-control has also played a vital role in maintaining social harmony and stability in Chinese society. The emphasis on self-restraint, respect for authority, and adherence to social norms has fostered a united social fabric and a sense of collective responsibility. Through exercising self-control in personal conduct and interactions, members contribute to the stability and well-being of their communities. This has ultimately contributed to the long-term stability and resilience of Chinese society. The concept of self-control has also been integral to the ideals of good governance and leadership in Chinese civilization.

Leaders and officials are expected to demonstrate self-discipline, restraint, and moral integrity in their actions and decision-making. This emphasis on self-control has played a crucial role in establishing trust, legitimacy, and continuity in governance. When leaders exhibit self-control, they contribute to effective governance and the enduring nature of Chinese political systems. Cultural traditions and rituals in China also place great importance on self-control. Practices like meditation, martial arts, calligraphy, and tea ceremonies encourage individuals to cultivate focus, mindfulness, and self-mastery. These cultural traditions not only promote personal well-being but also contribute to the preservation and transmission of Chinese cultural heritage across generations. They reinforce the value of self-control as a means to nurture personal virtues and maintain cultural continuity.

Moreover, self-control is closely linked to the long-term perspective that characterizes Chinese civilization. Chinese society has often demonstrated a forward-looking mindset when it comes to governance, economy, and societal development. This long-term perspective involves exercising self-control by prioritizing sustainable practices, planning for the future, and making present sacrifices for the benefit of future generations. This mindset has contributed to the resilience and longevity of Chinese civilization in the face of various challenges and transformations.

By placing emphasis on self-control, Chinese civilization has fostered social harmony, stability, cultural continuity, and a long-term perspective. It has played a significant role in shaping the endurance and longevity of Chinese civilization, positioning it as one of the world's oldest continuous civilizations.

Okinawan Civilization

Let's examine another case of civilization in our modern era where self-control and moderation have greatly influenced their long lifespan. The Okinawan population, renowned for their large number of centenarians and healthy aging, cannot solely attribute their longevity to practices of abstinence or celibacy. However, it can be attributed to regular practices of self-control and moderation, which are crucial aspects of celibacy and abstinence. The Okinawans have a cultural and historical background that places great importance on self-control, moderation, and mindfulness in various aspects of their lives, such as their diet and physical activities. While there is limited evidence directly linking celibacy or abstinence to their long lifespan, considering their religious practices reveals the significance of self-control and moderation.

Therefore, if we view celibacy and abstinence as outcomes of self-control and moderation, the evidence becomes overwhelming. Okinawan longevity is often associated with a combination of factors, including their traditional diet known as the "Okinawan diet," which is rich in vegetables, fruits, legumes, and fish. This diet is low in calories but high in nutrients, promoting good health and longevity. Additionally, the Okinawans foster a strong sense of community and social support networks, which contribute to their overall well-being and potentially have a positive impact on their longevity.

Moreover, the Okinawan people maintain a healthy lifestyle by engaging in various physical activities like walking, gardening, and participating in traditional martial arts such as karate. These active behaviors, along with their ability to reduce relationship stress and over-population, contribute to their overall health and longevity. It is worth noting that although sexual practices may differ among individuals within the Okinawan population, their emphasis on community, nutritious diet, physical exercise, and social connections are the primary factors associated with their extended lifespan. Abstaining from sexual activity or choosing celibacy, if practiced by some individuals, is likely a personal decision rather than a prevailing cultural norm or a definitive factor in their exceptional longevity. Their prolonged and healthy lives are generally attributed to a combination of factors, including maintaining a balanced diet, engaging in regular physical activity, having strong social support networks, and finding a sense of purpose in life, all of which involve self-control and moderation.

The Okinawan culture places great importance on moderation and self-control in different aspects of life, such as diet, physical activity, and overall lifestyle choices. However, it is difficult to draw firm conclusions about their sexual practices and how self-control in this area contributes to their long lifespan. It is crucial to acknowledge that discussions about sexual practices are intricate and can be influenced by various cultural, social, and personal factors. Additionally, there are numerous factors beyond sexual behavior that affect longevity, including diet, genetics, lifestyle choices, social connections, and environmental factors.

To truly understand the factors that contribute to the Okinawan population's long lifespan, comprehensive research is necessary, which should explore different facets of their lives, such as diet, social dynamics, healthcare, genetics, and overall lifestyle. Investigating the relationship between sexual practices, self-control, and longevity, specifically within the Okinawan context, requires detailed and culturally sensitive studies. While self-control and moderation are highly valued in Okinawan culture, making definitive claims about sexual practices or their direct impact on longevity is challenging.

The reasons behind the Okinawan population's long lifespan are diverse and involve various aspects of their lifestyles, social connections, diet, and cultural practices that go beyond sexual behaviors. To gain a comprehensive understanding of how religious practices affect sexual behavior, let's delve into their belief systems.

The majority of Okinawans follow a unique blend of indigenous religious beliefs called Ryukyuan religion or Ryukyuan spirituality. This spiritual tradition is exclusive to the Okinawan and Ryukyuan people and incorporates elements of animism, ancestor worship, and reverence for natural forces and spirits.

Ryukyuan religion places great importance on showing respect for ancestors through rituals and ceremonies that honor and pay tribute to them. The belief in kami, divine spirits, also holds significant prominence in Ryukyuan spirituality. These spirits are believed to reside within natural elements such as rocks, trees, and bodies of water. Additionally, Okinawa has a strong presence of Buddhism, with a considerable number of Okinawans practicing the Pure Land Buddhism sect. Pure Land Buddhism centers around the aspiration to be reborn in Amitabha Buddha's Pure Land, where enlightenment can be attained.

Furthermore, the religious landscape of Okinawa has been shaped by Shintoism, the native religion of

Japan. Many Okinawans incorporate Shinto practices and beliefs into their spiritual lives, such as visiting Shinto shrines and participating in related ceremonies.

It is important to recognize that Okinawa is a diverse region with a variety of religious beliefs and practices. While most Okinawans may follow Ryukyuan spirituality and incorporate elements of Buddhism and Shintoism, their religious affiliations can differ, including adherence to other faiths like Christianity or being non-religious. In the blue zone, where the majority of Okinawans reside, a blend of indigenous Ryukyuan spirituality, which includes animism and ancestor worship, is commonly practiced. Buddhism, particularly Pure Land Buddhism, and influences from Shintoism also hold significance in the religious landscape of Okinawa. Therefore, it is crucial to acknowledge the diverse religious beliefs and practices within the region, as individuals may have varying affiliations and expressions of spirituality.

Regarding the religious systems of Ryukyuan spirituality and Pure Land Buddhism, there may be variations in the specific rules and regulations related to sex and sexual behavior. It is important to note that the interpretation and application of these religious teachings can vary among individuals and communities, and there may not be universally agreed-upon guidelines.

In Ryukyuan spirituality, which is an indigenous belief system, there is no strict doctrine or set of rules specifically governing sexual behavior. Instead, the focus often lies on maintaining balance and harmony with nature, the community, and the spiritual realm. The practice of showing respect and reverence towards one's ancestors and the natural world is emphasized.

In Pure Land Buddhism, the emphasis typically lies on attaining enlightenment and liberation from the cycle of rebirth. Sexual behavior is generally guided by Buddhist ethical precepts, such as the Five Precepts, which provide guidelines for moral conduct.

These precepts include refraining from causing harm to living beings, refraining from taking what is not given, refraining from engaging in sexual misconduct, refraining from false speech, and refraining from consuming intoxicants.

When it comes to sexual behavior, the interpretation of "sexual misconduct" in Buddhism can vary. Generally, it includes actions like adultery, sexual violence, exploitation, and engaging in sexual activities that harm oneself or others. Buddhism encourages ethical and consensual sexual conduct, promoting relationships based on respect, mutual consent, and non-harm. However, it's important to recognize that different individuals may interpret and practice these teachings differently due to cultural norms, regional customs, and personal values.

Within Ryukyuan spirituality and Pure Land Buddhism, there are no specific rules solely dedicated to sexual behavior. Ryukyuan spirituality emphasizes harmony with nature and community, while Pure Land Buddhism promotes ethical conduct and non-harm. The details of sexual behavior within these traditions can vary, and individual beliefs and practices may be influenced by cultural, regional, and personal factors. To gain a more comprehensive understanding of specific teachings and practices within these traditions, it is advisable to consult local religious authorities or scholars.

Both Ryukyuan spirituality and Pure Land Buddhism consider self-control to be a fundamental aspect of their religious systems. Both traditions emphasize the cultivation of discipline and restraint as part of spiritual practice. In Ryukyuan spirituality, self-control is seen as crucial for maintaining harmony and balance within oneself, the community, and the natural world. It involves restraining desires and impulses and cultivating moderation and mindfulness in daily life. Self-control in this context encompasses various aspects, including emotions, behaviors, and interactions with others, all aimed at promoting harmony and spiritual well-being.

In the realm of Buddhism, including Pure Land Buddhism, the path of spiritual development heavily relies on self-control. Practicing self-control closely intertwines with adhering to ethical principles, which serve as a guide for moral behavior and the promotion of virtuous actions. Through exercising self-control, individuals refrain from engaging in harmful or unwholesome behaviors that may bring harm to themselves or others. Buddhism places great emphasis on nurturing self-control as a means to overcome mental impurities and reduce attachment, aversion, and delusion. It encourages the adoption of a disciplined approach to their thoughts, words, and actions, acknowledging the interconnected nature of their choices and the impact they have on themselves and others.

The development of self-control within these religious systems is often regarded as a pathway to personal growth, spiritual advancement, and the attainment of inner tranquility. It enables adherents to align their actions with their ethical and spiritual values, fostering a sense of integrity and inner harmony. However, it is crucial to understand that self-control should not be misconstrued as rigid suppression or denial of natural human instincts or desires. Rather, it involves cultivating mindfulness, awareness, and discernment to consciously make choices and act in ways that promote overall well-being, harmony, and spiritual growth.

In conclusion, self-control is widely recognized as an inherent element in the religious systems of Ryukyuan spirituality and Buddhism, including Pure Land Buddhism. It is viewed as a means to cultivate harmony, discipline, and moral conduct, thus facilitating personal growth and spiritual development. By nurturing self-control, we can align our actions with our values and contribute to our own well-being as well as the well-being of others. Interestingly, there is evidence suggesting that self-control is inherently passed down from one generation to the next, almost like an inherited gene.

Self-Control and Heredity

Scientific research has investigated the relationship between self-control and heredity, specifically examining the extent to which genetics may influence self-control abilities. It has been found that self-control is influenced by a combination of genetic and environmental factors. Studies have provided insights into the role of heredity in individual differences in self-control. Twin and family studies have been conducted to examine the heritability of self-control. These studies compare self-control measures among monozygotic (identical) and dizygotic (fraternal) twins to estimate the genetic contribution to self-control traits. The results suggest that genetic factors play a role in explaining some of the differences in self-control abilities.

Additionally, genetic association studies have aimed to identify specific genes associated with self-control. Large-scale genomic analyses have been conducted to identify variations in specific genes and their relationship to self-control outcomes. While this area of research is still ongoing, some studies have identified candidate genes that may be linked to self-control-related traits, such as genes related to dopamine functioning or neural pathways involved in impulse control. In other words, some people are born with a genetic trait that, upon expressing self-control, they experience a release of dopamine in relation to the delay of gratification, while others experience a release of dopamine upon the gratification of desire and other environmental factors in consideration. It is important to consider gene-environment interactions when examining the heredity of self-control.

Genetic influences on self-control interact with environmental factors. The expression of genetic predispositions may be influenced by environmental conditions and experiences. Factors such as parenting styles, socioeconomic status, and cultural influences shape the development and manifestation of self-control abilities. Gene-environment interactions contribute to the complex interplay between genetics and the environment in determining individual differences in self-control. Understanding the neuro-biological mechanisms underlying self-control has also provided insights into its potential genetic basis; however, it is very clear that the trait of self-restraint and dopamine reward is passed on to the next generation, as well as the lack of self-restraint and the subsequent rewards attached to that.

Neuro-imaging studies have identified brain regions and neural pathways associated with self-control processes. Genetic variations may impact the structure and functioning of these brain regions, influencing an individual's self-control abilities. The neuro-biological aspect of self-control offers further avenues for exploring the genetic underpinnings of self-control. It is important to note that self-control is a complex trait influenced by multiple factors, including genetic, environmental, and psychological factors.

Although scientific research indicates that there is a genetic aspect to self-control, it is important to acknowledge that self-control is a complex trait influenced by various factors. Genetic factors interact with environmental and psychological factors to shape the differences in self-control abilities among individuals. More research is necessary to enhance our understanding of the genetic foundations of self-control and how they interact with environmental influences to shape this significant characteristic. Similarly, celibacy and abstinence encounter different challenges and misconceptions that can affect those who choose to adopt these practices.

Chapter 10: Overcoming Challenges and Misunderstandings

The practices of celibacy and abstinence have faced numerous challenges and misconceptions due to societal norms and expectations. One particular challenge that individuals who choose celibacy and abstinence may encounter is the pressure and expectations imposed by society regarding sexual activity. In a culture that often prioritizes sexual experiences and relationships as the norm, those who opt for celibacy or abstinence may face scrutiny, misunderstanding, or judgment from others who do not share their values or beliefs. It is crucial to acknowledge that misconceptions about celibacy and abstinence can arise from a lack of understanding about the reasons behind these practices.

Misunderstandings often revolve around the false notion that those practicing celibacy or abstinence are repressed, uninterested in sex, or incapable of finding a partner. However, the decision to embrace celibacy or abstinence is frequently a personal choice driven by various factors, such as spirituality, personal values, health considerations, personal growth, or the desire to establish emotional connections before engaging in sexual activity. The limited awareness of the potential benefits of celibacy and abstinence contributes to these misconceptions.

In reality, these practices offer individuals opportunities for personal growth, self-discovery, emotional well-being, and the development of deeper non-sexual connections. However, the purpose and value of celibacy and abstinence are often misunderstood or overlooked.

Challenges of Practicing Celibacy and Abstinence

Unrealistic expectations of perfection can pose challenges for those practicing celibacy and abstinence. Some may hold unrealistic expectations that individuals practicing celibacy or abstinence should flawlessly commit to their choices and never experience any sexual desires or struggles. However, it is important to recognize that celibacy and abstinence are personal journeys that come with their own set of challenges and occasional moments of temptation. Difficulties along the way are normal, and personal growth is an ongoing process.

The lack of support and understanding can be a significant challenge for those practicing celibacy and abstinence. Finding a supportive community or those who share similar values and choices can also be difficult. This lack of open conversations or societal acceptance can lead to feelings of isolation or being misunderstood. Having a support system of like-minded people or access to resources is crucial in navigating the challenges and misconceptions associated with celibacy and abstinence. These challenges and misconceptions stem from societal expectations, limited awareness, unrealistic expectations, and lack of support. Recognizing and addressing these challenges and misconceptions can promote understanding, respect, and empathy for those who choose celibacy and abstinence as personal lifestyle choices.

Another significant challenge is managing sexual desires and temptations. Suppressing or redirecting these natural and instinctual desires can be difficult, leading to internal conflicts.

Additionally, the dedication and self-discipline required for celibacy or abstinence can be demanding. This lifestyle choice involves resisting temptations, navigating challenging situations, and finding alternative ways to fulfill emotional and physical needs. Staying true to one's decision may require regular self-reflection, perseverance, and support from like-minded individuals. However, those who practice celibacy or abstinence may also face challenges such as loneliness and the longing for companionship or intimacy.

Choosing celibacy or abstinence can sometimes lead to feelings of isolation or a sense of missing out on experiences that others may be enjoying. The desire for emotional connection and companionship may persist, and we may need to find alternative ways to fulfill these needs, such as building strong friendships or engaging in meaningful, non-sexual relationships.

Furthermore, navigating relationships and dating while practicing celibacy or abstinence can present its own set of challenges. It is important to communicate one's choices and boundaries to potential partners and establish compatible relationships that align with one's values. This may require open and honest communication, finding partners who share similar values or are understanding of one's choices, and being mindful of emotional and physical boundaries.

Strategies to Overcome the Challenges of Celibacy and Abstinence

Adopting celibacy or practicing abstinence can come with various difficulties, including managing sexual desires, facing social pressures and expectations, maintaining consistency and commitment, dealing with feelings of loneliness or longing, and navigating relationships. It is crucial for us to be aware of these potential challenges and find strategies, support systems, and coping mechanisms that can help us navigate and overcome these difficulties on our chosen path of celibacy or abstinence.

In order to overcome the difficulties of choosing celibacy or practicing abstinence, it is crucial to possess resilience, self-reflection, and supportive methods. Take the time to deeply contemplate your motivations and values for selecting this path. Gain clarity on why it holds significance to you and reaffirm your commitment. This self-awareness will strengthen our determination and help us remain focused on our objectives despite the challenges. Surround ourselves with others who share similar values and join supportive communities. Connecting with like-minded people who understand and respect our choices can provide invaluable support, encouragement, and a sense of belonging.

Engage in conversations, exchange experiences, and learn from others who are on a similar journey. Communicate openly with friends, family, and potential partners about your choices. Clear and honest communication can manage expectations, foster understanding, and cultivate respect. Find healthy outlets to manage sexual desires and temptations, such as engaging in exercise, meditation, hobbies, or pursuing personal passions. Cultivate deep emotional connections with others, develop meaningful friendships, and invest in building strong emotional bonds. Prioritize self-care and emotional well-being through activities like self-reflection, journaling, therapy, mindfulness, or relaxation techniques.

It is important that we stay mindful of our choices and be open to adapting as challenges arise. Educate yourself about the benefits and reasons behind celibacy or abstinence. Remember that each person's journey is unique, so discover strategies that resonate with you personally. Be patient, celebrate your progress, and seek support when necessary. By possessing resilience, self-awareness, and supportive methods, you can navigate the challenges and find fulfillment on your chosen path.

Chapter 11:
Modern Perspectives on Celibacy and Abstinence

While celibacy and abstinence have historical and religious origins, they are also viewed through a contemporary lens. In today's society, people are considering celibacy and abstinence as deliberate lifestyle choices influenced by various factors, including personal development, health, the environment, and cultural shifts. Here is an overview of some modern perspectives on celibacy and abstinence.

I believe many people see celibacy and abstinence as conscious choices that can allow us to prioritize personal growth and self-discovery; however, our challenge is taking action in an environment where we are continuously bombarded with cultural and media messages telling us to live otherwise. By abstaining from sexual activity from time to time, we can redirect our energy towards other aspects of life, such as education, career advancement, pursuing personal interests, and maintaining emotional well-being. Embracing celibacy or abstinence will provide an opportunity for us to explore our own identity, values, and goals without the distractions or pressures associated with sexual relationships.

Another contemporary perspective on celibacy and abstinence is driven by health considerations. People may choose to abstain from sexual activity to prioritize their physical and mental well-being. This perspective recognizes that engaging in sexual activity carries potential risks such as sexually transmitted infections (STIs) or emotional complications. By practicing celibacy or abstinence, we can minimize these risks and focus on maintaining overall health and well-being.

In recent years, an increasing number of us have adopted practices meant to preserve the environment; however, we may see celibacy or abstinence as a response to environmental concerns, as the habit of being led by our passions and desires pulls us away from choosing celibacy and abstinence as a choice too. Recognizing the impact of overpopulation on the planet's resources and ecological balance, some people choose to limit their reproductive contributions by abstaining from sexual activity or committing to long-term celibacy, but the impact of these few is minimal. This growing perspective reflects a slow awakening to the fact that our free love sexual behavior can no longer sustain a healthy planet. To create a future where human life is sustainable and to minimize our carbon footprint, taking into account the broader implications of continuing to follow our current sexual behavior, we must weigh the global implications of this on population growth.

Contemporary perspectives on celibacy and abstinence also highlight the significance of personal empowerment and autonomy. Opting to abstain from sexual activity can be an act of self-empowerment, enabling individuals to take control over their own bodies, desires, and boundaries. It can also provide us with focus so that we can build wealth we can use to build a culture that sustains our planet rather than destroys it. It upholds the idea that we have the right to define their own sexual experiences and engage in consensual activities based on their own values and comfort levels apart from the "free love and drug use" values of our parents, the Baby Boomers and the culture and industries they created.

Furthermore, some modern perspectives emphasize the positive impact of celibacy and abstinence on reshaping relationship dynamics and fostering deeper emotional connections. I am sure many of us who put physical intimacy above emotional intimacy know all too well the separation, pain, and trauma this brought us. By refraining from physical intimacy for period of time, we can prioritize emotional intimacy and establish strong connections built on shared values, emotional support, and genuine communication. This perspective challenges the notion we have been taught by the choices and actions of the previous generation that physical intimacy is the sole foundation of a fulfilling relationship, emphasizing the importance of emotional connection, mutual understanding, and shared goals.

It is worth noting once more that contemporary perspectives on celibacy and abstinence vary greatly among individuals. The motivations and reasons for choosing these practices are diverse and personal. Some may temporarily embrace celibacy or abstinence as a period of self-reflection, while others may commit to lifelong abstinence due to their beliefs or values. These contemporary perspectives reflect the ever-changing societal attitudes toward sexuality and personal choices. Embracing celibacy or abstinence in today's world is considered a valid and respected choice, rooted in our autonomy, self-care, personal growth, and alignment with personal values and aspirations.

Chapter 12:
Harnessing the Power of Celibacy and Abstinence for Financial Growth

The mental and physical health benefits of celibacy and abstinence are closely intertwined with the opportunities they provide for personal development and goal achievement. Personally, abstaining from sex has allowed me to prevent unintended pregnancy and the risk of sexually transmitted infections (STIs). This preventive aspect not only contributes to my physical well-being but also frees me from the potential stress and health concerns associated with sexual activity and the benefits of that.

Furthermore, celibacy and abstinence afford me the mental clarity and focus needed to direct my attention toward personal goals and aspirations. This heightened clarity and focus have enabled me to pursue educational endeavors, advance in my career, and prioritize my mental health with unwavering determination. The absence of distractions related to sexual activity has created a space for me to channel my energy and attention into my ambitions, fostering a sense of purpose and drive that propels me toward achieving my goals.

Moreover, the enhanced character traits that celibacy can foster, such as restraint, patience, and self-compassion, as mentioned by Verywell Mind, have contributed to the development of a strong foundation for goal achievement. Restraint and patience are essential virtues that have enabled me to stay committed to my long-term objectives, even in the face of challenges or setbacks. The clarity of mind obtained through celibacy has helped me cultivate a deep understanding of my personal values and aspirations, providing a clear road map for my journey toward success. This mental clarity has allowed me to make well-informed decisions, set meaningful goals, and stay focused on my chosen path. With a clear vision of my aspirations and an unwavering focus on my goals, I have been able to harness the transformative power of celibacy and abstinence to achieve remarkable personal and professional accomplishments.

The mental and emotional well-being that celibacy and abstinence have afforded me is truly transformative. With a clear mind and a deep sense of emotional balance, I have been able to approach challenges with resilience and optimism. This emotional equilibrium has allowed me to navigate the complexities of personal and professional life with a sense of calm and confidence, contributing to my overall well-being and success. As Norman Vincent Peale once said, "Change your thoughts, and you change your world." This quote resonates deeply with me, as it reflects the profound impact of mental and emotional well-being on our ability to shape our lives and achieve our aspirations.

In embracing celibacy and abstinence, I have found an inner strength and resilience that has bolstered my mental and emotional well-being. This has translated into a heightened capacity to cope with stress, overcome obstacles, and maintain a positive outlook even in the face of adversity. The newfound mental clarity has empowered me to make sound decisions, set meaningful goals, and pursue personal growth with a deep sense of purpose. Additionally, the emotional stability I have gained has enhanced my relationships, both personally and professionally, fostering a greater sense of empathy, understanding, and connection with others.

The mental and emotional well-being that celibacy and abstinence have cultivated within me has been instrumental in shaping my personal and professional journey. With a clear mind, emotional balance, and unwavering determination, I am better equipped to pursue my passions, achieve my goals, and make a positive impact on the world around me.

Moreover, the clarity and energy gained have instilled in me a profound sense of purpose. I have found myself driven by a deep conviction to make a positive impact in the world, leveraging my newfound clarity and focus to contribute meaningfully to causes that align with my values. This heightened sense of purpose has fueled my motivation to engage in activities that promote well-being, sustainability, and positive change. It has inspired me to seek out opportunities where I can use my skills, resources, and influence to create a lasting, positive impact on the world around me.

This profound sense of purpose has permeated every aspect of my life, influencing my interactions with others, my approach to decision-making, and my commitment to personal growth. It has driven me to seek out opportunities for positive change, both in my own life and in the world around me. With a clear vision and a deep sense of purpose, I am committed to making meaningful contributions to the well-being of others and the sustainability of our planet.

The transformative power of celibacy and abstinence has empowered me to live a purpose-driven life filled with passion, determination, and a commitment to positive change. These qualities have become the guiding principles that shape my personal and professional journey, propelling me toward a future characterized by meaningful achievements and a deep sense of fulfillment.

Embracing a lifestyle of celibacy or abstinence has provided me with the mental clarity and energy needed to delve into entrepreneurial ventures such as multi-level marketing (MLM). The discipline and focus cultivated through celibacy have been channeled toward building a successful MLM business. With a clear vision and heightened determination, I leverage the principles of MLM to generate wealth and financial independence. It's important to note that the rewards of MLM take time and effort, but with persistence and a clear goal in mind, backed by the benefits we obtain from our practice of celibacy and/or abstinence, the potential for financial success is within reach.

There is no other endeavor available today that can transport anyone with focus, drive, clarity, determination, and passion to multimillionaire status like multi-level marketing. The key is to find the right company whose product has the most impact on your life. Align with successful persons within and do exactly what they do and tell you to do. The wealth we generate through successful MLM endeavors can be utilized to support initiatives aimed at creating a sustainable future for the planet. When you have embraced celibacy or abstinence, the focus you gain blazes a brilliant light, illuminating your path to wealth generation through passive income.

It frees you to pursue personal interests such as global change, investing in businesses, and developing new technologies. This financial freedom allows you to contribute to environmental conservation efforts, renewable energy projects, and innovative technologies for sustainable living.

Multi-level marketing levels the playing field, providing an opportunity for the average person with little or no education to become a multimillionaire, thereby empowering individuals to make a significant impact on the world.

With the financial means derived from your successful MLM venture, you can reinvest in other enterprises, research, and development of new technologies that promote environmental sustainability and life-giving solutions, or travel and teach others how to do exactly as you. You may become involved in funding green technology startups, supporting scientific research in fields such as renewable energy and conservation, and collaborating with like-minded individuals to drive innovation for a sustainable and thriving Earth. Through your dedication to celibacy or abstinence until you begin to experience the fruits of it, one of the those fruits being a profound sense of clarity and a hunger for knowledge with which you can change yourself and play an active role in shaping a better future, you will experience transformation that leads to wealth in every form if you stick with it. With your new mind and new wealth you can invest in making your community and the world a better place.

Chapter 13:
Join the Activation Nation

Dr. Joe M. McCord, a world-renowned professor of biochemistry, discovered the enzyme superoxide dismutase (SOD) while a graduate student under fellow redox pioneer Irwin Fridovich. Superoxide dismutase (SOD) is an important antioxidant enzyme that helps to neutralize free radicals in the body, which can cause damage to cells and contribute to aging and various diseases. In his book, "The Quest for Life," Dr. Sanjay Gupta explores the concept of functional aging, focusing on extending a healthy and active life. The book delves into the impact of SOD in extending one's healthy and active life.

The phrase "activation nation" refers to those who take the supplement Protandim, a nutritional supplement comprised of five plant extracts (milk thistle, bacopa, ashwagandha root, turmeric, green tea) that activate the Nuclear factor (nrf) pathway that is integral to several antioxidant enzymes which capture and dispose of aging and disease-causing free-radicals. Protandim, a patented formula, has been shown to have a positive effect on the production of superoxide dismutase (SOD).

Studies have demonstrated that Protandim, a nutraceutical consisting of a combination of medicinal plants, can induce superoxide dismutase (SOD) and catalase activities. This induction of SOD and catalase activities is associated with a reduction in superoxide generation and lipid peroxidation in healthy human subjects. The findings suggest that Protandim can contribute to the enhancement of antioxidant defense mechanisms in the body. Those who take the supplement on a regular basis are said to be "activated."

When a person is activated, it simply means the body is producing 40% more anti-aging enzymes than the average person who is declining in the production of SOD and Catalase. According to a study published in the National Center for Biotechnology Information, increasing SOD production can contribute to en-hanced antioxidant defense mechanisms in the body, potentially reducing oxidative stress and its associ-ated damage.

This reduction in oxidative stress may have positive effects on overall health and could potentially con-tribute to the aging process. Another study published in a scientific journal indicates that a significant in-crease in SOD activity can help prevent oxidative stress and damage, which are fundamental in a vari-ety of disease pathologies. This suggests that a 40% increase in SOD production may contribute to the prevention of oxidative stress-related diseases.

Additionally, research has shown that decreased SOD expression increases vulnerability to oxidative stress. Therefore, an increase in SOD production could potentially help protect against the damaging effects of oxidative stress and contribute to overall health and well-being. In summary, a 40% increase in SOD production may lead to enhanced antioxidant defense mechanisms, reduced oxidative stress, and potentially contribute to overall health and aging by protecting against oxidative stress-related damage. Essentially, in my words, our cells are restored to function like those of our younger selves. After about 30 days on the product, depending on your physiology with results varying, you are ACTIVATED! How does this relate to celibacy and abstinence?

Combining the use of Protandim as part of an overall lifestyle change that incorporates exercise and diet changes can have a profound impact overall health. I believe that along with the use of Protandim combined with periods of abstinence or celibacy, we may potentially have an even greater impact on our overall health, particularly in relation to emotional and oxidative stress reduction. Protandim is known to promote the production of superoxide dismutase

(SOD), which plays a key role in defending against free radicals and reducing oxidative stress, a common by-product of cellular respiration.

Abstinence and celibacy, when practiced consciously, may lead to reduced exposure to certain diseases and can contribute to lower emotional and mental stress associated with sexual activity. The potential reduction in emotional stress could indirectly contribute to lower oxidative stress, as emotional stress is known to be a factor in the body's overall oxidative burden.

While I only have anecdotal evidence that suggests that using Protandim and my choice to practice abstinence have had health benefits for me, it's important to note that the effects of these practices on overall health are multifaceted and can vary from person to person. It's always advisable to consult with a healthcare professional before making significant changes to one's lifestyle or adding new supplements to one's routine.

Conclusion

In conclusion, "Change Yourself, Change the World: Harness Your Sexual Energy for Activation" provides a comprehensive exploration of the multifaceted impact of celibacy and abstinence on individuals and society at large. The journey through the book takes readers on an enlightening path, from addressing immediate concerns such as decreasing crime rates and preventing the transmission of STDs to broader and more far-reaching effects like population reduction and global impact.

The historical origins of celibacy and abstinence are thoughtfully examined, shedding light on the cultural and societal foundations of these practices. The advantages of adopting celibacy and abstinence are outlined, not only in terms of personal well-being but also in their positive contributions to the social and economic fabric of communities.

The book emphasizes the essential connection between self-control and societal well-being, illustrating how individual choices can ripple through the collective consciousness. It explores the challenges and misunderstandings associated with celibacy and abstinence, offering insights on how to overcome them in a modern context.

Furthermore, the financial growth potential associated with harnessing the power of celibacy and abstinence is explored in-depth. Readers are encouraged to join the "Activation Nation," a community dedicated to leveraging sexual energy for personal transformation and wealth-building. The final chapter serves as a call to action, urging readers to spread the message of sexual energy for holistic transformation, wealth creation, and societal activation.

In crafting this enlightening and thought-provoking book, the author invites readers to reconsider their relationship with their own sexuality and, in doing so, contributes to a broader dialogue about personal responsibility, societal well-being, and the potential for positive change. "Change Yourself, Change the World" challenges conventional perspectives, offering a compelling vision of how the mindful harnessing of sexual energy can be a catalyst for individual and collective growth, ultimately paving the way for a more activated and harmonious world.

References

Geng, Y., Gu, J., Wang, J., & Zhang, R. (2021). Smartphone addiction and depression, anxiety: The role of bedtime procrastination and self-control. Journal of Affective Disorders, 293, 415–421. https://doi.org/10.1016/j.jad.2021.06.062

Cartledge, P. (2004). The Spartans: The World of the Warrior-Heroes of Ancient Greece. Vintage.

Willems, Y. E., Boesen, N., Li, J., Finkenauer, C., & Bartels, M. (2019). The heritability of self-control: A meta-analysis. Neuroscience and biobehavioral reviews, 100, 324–334. https://doi.org/10.1016/j.neubiorev.2019.02.012

Buettner, D. (2010). The Blue Zones: Lessons for Living Longer from the People Who've Lived the Longest. United States: National Geographic Society.

Arnold, C. (2004). Easter Island: Giant Stone Statues Tell of a Rich and Tragic Past. United States: CLARION BOOKS.

Gibbon, E. (2013). History of the Decline and Fall of the Roman Empire Vol 1. United States: Start Publishing LLC.

"Reproductive Rituals in Ancient Mesoamerica" by Vera Tiesler and Andrea Cucina

"Sexual Ideology and the Fall of Classic Maya Civilization" by Richard G. Lesure

"Sexual Magic and Fertility Rituals in Ancient Maya Society" by Nikolai Grube

"The Role of Women in Ancient Maya Society: Pregnancy, Childbirth, and Postpartum Care" by Amanda M. Harvey

Olsen, J. A., Weed, S. E., Ritz, G. M., & Jensen, L. C. (1991). The Effects of Three Abstinence Sex Education Programs On Student Attitudes Toward Free Radical Biology & Medicine, Vol. 5, pp. 363-369, 1988 0891-5849/88 $3.00 + .00 Printed in the USA. All rights reserved. © 1988 Pergamon Press plc

McCord JM, Fridovich I (November 1969). "Superoxide dismutase. An enzymic function for erythrocuprein (hemocuprein)". *J. Biol. Chem.* 244 (22): 6049–55. doi:10.1016/S0021-9258(18)63504-5. PMID 5389100.

Keele BB, McCord JM, Fridovich I (November 1970). "Superoxide dismutase from escherichia coli B. A new manganese-containing enzyme". *J. Biol. Chem.* 245 (22): 6176–81. doi:10.1016/S0021-9258(18)62675-4. PMID 4921969.

Free Radical Biology and Medicine, Volume 17, Issue 3, September 1994, Pages 249-258

PLoS One. 2009; 4(4): e5284. Published online 2009 Apr 22. doi: 10.1371/journal.pone.0005284

PMCID: PMC2668769PMID: 19384424

Protandim, a Fundamentally New Antioxidant Approach in Chemoprevention Using Mouse Two-Stage Skin Carcinogenesis as a Model Jianfeng Liu, [1] Xin Gu, [2] Delira Robbins, [1] Guohong Li, [3] Runhua Shi, [4] Joe M. McCord, [5] and Yunfeng Zhao[1]

J Diet Suppl. Author manuscript; available in PMC 2010 Aug 24.*Published in final edited form as:* J Diet Suppl. 2010 Jun 1; 7(2): 159–178. doi: 10.3109/19390211.2010.482041. PMCID: PMC2926985NIHMSID: NIHMS226268PMID: 20740052

The Dietary Supplement Protandim® Decreases Plasma Osteopontin and Improves Markers of Oxidative Stress in Muscular Dystrophy *Mdx* Mice. Muhammad Muddasir Qureshi, MD, MPH, Warren C. McClure, MS, Nicole L.

Arevalo, MA, Rick E. Rabon, BA, Benjamin Mohr, Swapan K. Bose, BS, BPharm, Joe M. McCord, PhD, and Brian S. Tseng, MD, PhD

PLoS One. 2010 Jul 30;5(7):e11902. doi: 10.1371/journal.pone.0011902. The chemopreventive effects of Protandim: modulation of p53 mitochondrial translocation and apoptosis during skin carcinogenesis. Delira Robbins 1, Xin Gu, Runhua Shi, Jianfeng Liu, Fei Wang, Jacqulyne Ponville, Joe M McCord, Yunfeng Zhao

About the Author

Floyd Jones Sanders is the Principal and Managing Director at P.A.C.E. Family Services, an agency providing anger parenting, anger management Counseling, and Exchange services in California. Floyd graduated from UC Davis with a degree in Analytic Philosophy and History. He is a professional anger management counselor, certified Domestic Violence therapist, and Life Coach. He is certified in the ABCs of Parenting through Yale University. Floyd has over 25 years of experience in the field of individual counseling, coaching, and family services.

He currently lives in Sacramento, California. If you would like more information about coaching/counseling services or the network marketing company

Floyd is a part of, or you are interested in becoming a distributor or customer, see the contact information information below.

www.pacefamilyservices.com

www.floydsanders.lifevantage.com

email: floydj.sanders@outlooklook.com